GOOD COP
GOOD COP

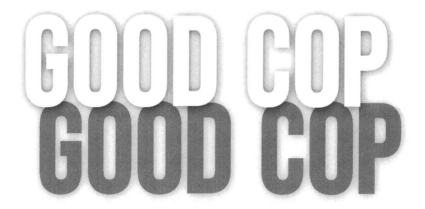

A Get Healthy, Stay Healthy Guide for Law Enforcement

Brian Casey

ALLEY LIGHT PRESS
Saint Paul, Minnesota

Alley Light Press
Saint Paul, Minnesota
editor@alleylightpress.com
www.alleylightpress.com

Library of Congress Control Number: 2018953960

Editing by Jean Cook and Maureen Johnson.
Book design by David Farr of ImageSmythe.
Printed by Bookmobile
Printed in the United States of America on acid-free paper.

ISBN 978-1-7325651-0-4

First Printing, 2018

CONTENTS

To my wife and children, who know best the heart of a cop.

To the cops working at this very moment,
who act as guardians to defend, protect and provide,
willingly occupying the space between order and disorder.

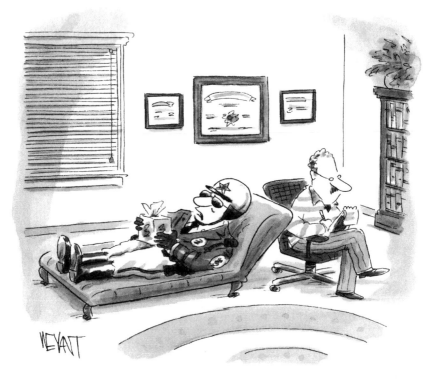

"Sometimes I can't remember if I'm good cop or bad cop."

"To Do and to Bear is the Duty of Life"

— Unknown

P OLICE WORK MUST HAVE HAD ITS ORIGINS from the time when humans first gathered in groups. A trustworthy and able-bodied member of the group was selected to keep watch and protect the others from danger while they slept. Eventually as societies grew, the duty evolved to an occupation with the night watchman calling out "All's well." People lived better because they knew, as they do today if they pause to consider it, "We sleep peacefully in our beds at night only because rough men [and women] stand ready to do violence on our behalf."[1]

Recently, I attended a conference on the subject of psychological trauma. Every day, every lecture, I thought, *Save Yourself,* and wrote the words like a heading at the top of each page of notes. A lot can go wrong in life, and we are foolish to put our welfare exclusively in the hands of others, even the so-called experts. Our health, our family's wellbeing, and our positive contribution to the functionality of the police force, require self-awareness, self-examination and self-determination. While police work depends wonderfully on interdependence, good street cops know they must keep their mind and body right, remaining prepared to prevail alone in a bloody fight to the death.

As a patrol officer, when assigned a civilian ride-along, I gave my rider the same Save Yourself warning. If they wanted to get close to the action, I would try to get them close, but warned them to be careful, not to stand there flat-footed and get punched in the face because they were waiting for me to tell them to duck.

We have our own version of flat-footedness as cops, when we figuratively blame others for our bloody nose or lie on the floor and moan, "Fix me." Some of the best help is the help we seek, desire, or orchestrate for ourselves. A friend in recovery told me the best things that happened to him were generated by him. And if you are in a bad way, feeling lost, unsure, and without a plan, saving yourself can include asking for help from a friend or professional. We should not pretend that good help is unavailable, it is usually only a phone call away. Self-help resources are within arm's reach, and honest self-reflection is immediately available and waiting. This book can be a means of saving yourself starting with a better understanding of what I call Cop Think™.

The Work

We live in a remarkably orderly society, but we suspect it would rapidly deteriorate without the police keeping watch. While at the same time, we might marvel at how little control we actually have or how often a very few of us maintain a facade of control. Today the police, men and women of probably mostly average intelligence and not a lot of formal education, maintain or restore order and enforce some of the rules and laws of the land. We say "No" to people. "No, you can't park on the sidewalk." "No, you can't beat your spouse." "No, you can't take other people's stuff." And we deal with *no people,* those who say "no" with their words or actions to even simple requests or lawful orders, no matter how they are phrased or delivered.

This only works because of the understanding, threat if you will, that there is a potential for violence, the preferred term would be force, "police force." Back when some cops still carried revolvers, I witnessed a New Orleans cop single-handedly push back an angry crowd of about 200 people. He first pushed the front of his squad into the mob getting their full attention and signaling that he might be crazy. Then he leapt out with his nightstick loaded under his arm and leaned forward barking and snarling like a mad dog. It only worked because of his threat of violence, and how convincingly he signaled his readiness to use it. We are now in the time of probably the best-behaved police officers in the history of policing, and force is rarely used, but like it or not, our job remains workable only with the possibility of force behind it. We are good at our jobs and must keep our authority legitimate so we can be effective. With our kindness in plain view and our fierceness partially concealed, we can go about the business of keeping order and watching out for trouble.

Police work is a job like no other, for some a vocation or a calling. But it is a job where another cop can be put in your place if you are not there. Feeling chosen is virtuous, but not a requirement. The police department is primarily a workplace where the first priority is the work that needs to be done, not the needs of individual workers. If we get this backwards it becomes chaos and neither goal is met. As workers, we have both an individual and shared purpose and function which includes both running towards danger and numerous mundane tasks. We must do all of our work well.

At the time of this writing, I am a police sergeant and the director of the department's Employee Assistance Program (EAP). In that role, I may see the police department like no one else does. From my perspective, probably the single best thing an agency can do to support the mental health and wellbeing of its police officers, is to have a high-functioning police department, independent of mental health and wellness resources. A high-functioning department provides clarity of purpose and, where possible, reduces stress by decreasing uncertainty and increasing predictability. Each and every employee of the police department has a role in this. Cops deal in disorder in the street, they need stable ground on which to stand, especially during times of great flux, with a *few* clear expectations that are well communicated and consistently attended to.

To effectively help troubled cops in the workplace, one must be both compassionate and strategic. If you have to choose one, I would say be strategic. Caring for all cops includes holding them accountable to work expectations and acting deliberately to correct poor work behavior. The troubled cop, whether he is an alcoholic or a malcontent, not only harms himself but may also harm the organization. Trying to correct his behavior can demand an enormous amount of supervisory time and attention. This energy is not unlimited, and one of the greatest disservices we do in the workplace is to under serve the earnest employee while we are busy attending to problem people. The earnest cops are the ones that show up on time, do not ask for special favors and quietly go about the work as constant contributors. The workplace is like a living organism that needs to sustain the earnest cop and protect itself from the ravages of a troubled cop.

Evidence

I have tried to cite evidence to back up the material within this book, and I believe I did so with some success. However, some statements are based solely on my observations and experience, which is vulnerable to interpretation and occasional magical thinking. In other words, I might be wrong, and in some places, repeating unchallenged assumptions.

This is not a homicide investigation where evidence is everything. In some places *Good Cop, Good Cop* is more like a confession. However, we know that some confessions are false, or the homicides are justified. Evidence has a few down sides as well. It takes time to gather; sometimes the evidence is misleading or gathered to support one view while other evidence is ignored that supports a contrary view. And evidence is always looking backwards.

As we know in police work, misinformation can be more dangerous than no information, and we should be on guard. Do cops have a higher rate of divorce or suicide? It is not so clear or may not be true. And is a higher rate even important when due to self-selection and careful job screening, we start out healthier than the general population? The better questions might be, do we make divorce easier for cops? Does suicide risk for retired or command staff go unnoticed despite the fact that white males between the ages of 45 and 64 take their own lives more than any other group.[2,3] Just as when you are responding to a call and dispatch broadcasts that there are "No weapons in the house" or "He won't fight with the police," you should come to your own conclusions, and compare things to your own experience and observations.

I will no doubt appear to contradict myself, either because I lack some clarity myself or because clarity within complexity appears contradictory and messy. *Good Cop, Good Cop* attempts to speak to one of the most interesting creatures I know, the police officer. And although being too differential to our uniqueness can interfere with healthy normalization or further estrangement from society, I do recognize that police officers stand alone in society as both citizen and guardian.

"Cop"

I will use the word, cop or police officer throughout this book. Generally, "cop" when talking as if to another cop, and "police officer" when speaking as if to a general audience. I prefer the word police officer then because it denotes, for me, a higher level of respect. For simplicity, I will not use the term law enforcement, but the audience I am thinking of are all those who wear the badge and carry the gun, the rough men and women who keep watch over others.

The intended reader of this book is primarily the police officer and sometimes includes those who supervise officers or command an agency. The messages intended for the officer may also be useful to those who love a police officer, or professionals who assist officers in mental or emotional distress. While writing each chapter I continuously visualized cops as I know them, because I am a cop and have been a longtime observer of cops. I do not view cops as heroes or villains, saviors or victims. Just laborers who are occasionally sick, injured or confused about what it means to be a good cop. Or maybe they feel as if they have been living with a low-grade fever of sorts and not feeling well. Personal struggles are often unavoidable, sometimes necessary. If we are to act heroically, let us right ourselves, *save ourselves*. If we act as saviors, let it be to demonstrate our own health in how well we live and to reach out to other cops in distress.

PART I

HEALTH AND WELLBEING

W E WANT TO THINK WELL, FEEL WELL AND MOVE WELL, have a
sound body and mind. Wellness requires giving time and attention
to doing things that are good for us while avoiding, minimizing, or recovering from the things that are bad or harm us. This might be simply stated,
but it is not always so simply applied to our lives as we struggle with things
like stress, fitness and adequate sleep.

It is important that we point ourselves in the right direction. In my
public safety career, I have more than once driven the wrong way in a
hurry, with red lights and siren. The first step, the moment you suspect you
are on the wrong route, is to shut off the emergency equipment, then slow
down or stop.

It might be tempting to think of health and wellbeing as something
that happens to us instead of something we choose. The term locus of
control refers to the degree to which a person believes he has control over
the outcome of his life. Those with an internal locus of control do better in
all areas of health and wellbeing, and it is central to resiliency.[1] Without an
internal locus of control, we can end up going the wrong way fast.

I recognize there is harm from the experience of police work, but I
reject the idea that the job ruins us. Instead, if we feel ruined, we may
have failed to find and update our personal mission or purpose as a police
officer; or we have been unable or unwilling to face the hardships we

brought with us to the job; or we have simply been inattentive to our health and wellbeing. The next few chapters focus on some of the fundamentals of good health, increasing our physical activity, improving our nutrition, managing our thinking and improving our sleep.

Police work can be difficult, but so is working in sales, being a teacher, roofing houses, or anything you commit to doing well. Police work is the work we chose, and there are many advantages to being a cop. It is our responsibility to make sure we are going in the right direction toward our best health and wellbeing.

CHAPTER 1

COP THINK

Why the Police Do What They Do

Cops Are Smart — They Study Humans

Cops are smart in ways that I admire a great deal; they study the world and human behavior for a living. My father, who was a salesman, had a knack for this. I first recognized it as a small child; we were driving along when we approached two people standing near the roadway on the shoulder. He suddenly put both hands on the wheel and jerked the car to give them extra room. When I asked what had happened, he said, "That one guy bent over to pick up something off the ground, when people do that and stand up again, they sometimes take a step to the right or left."

As a young paramedic, I watched a group of officers at their best. I had just declared a woman dead after she had been shot on Christmas day by her ex-husband. Out on the sidewalk, the current husband was wild with want. I could not bear to face the man and instead addressed one of the officers saying simply, "She's dead." The officer turned to the man and explained to him that his wife could not be saved. The man began to wail and to strikeout at the air. I was frightened that he would attack me, and I moved off onto the lawn. The officers formed a circle around him, keeping their posture loose without suggesting an offensive. Their bodies, the posts, and their arms, the ropes, of a boxing ring. He moved from officer to officer, striking their chests and rolled off their arms. He weakened as they called out, "Let it out man. Let it out." His unobstructed hysteria slowly gave way to crying, then sobbing. He stood with his head down and his shoulders slack, in the center of the ring. I never admired a group of men more than I did these police officers in that moment; they were masters of their craft with talents for things most of us did not know were needed.

Survival

The transition to cop requires a rapid shedding of naivete as we try, both successfully and unsuccessfully, to be as rough and tough as the rough and tough world we police.[1] Over time, this can leave some feeling lonely and misunderstood or with a vague sense that something is not right with them, that they are defective or damaged. Additionally, society's mixed messages to and about cops can be very confusing and make things worse. Society says it prefers gentle men and women, who with sympathetic faces, listen well and nod their understanding, but they also ask for them to be able and willing to bust down a door or put a bullet in someone's ear. Society cannot always have it both ways, though some demand it.

I am not suggesting that officers cannot and should not be friendly, in fact they should be, it is part of service. But society might need to know what I had in my locker, next to the picture of my wife and kids, my own version of General James Mattis's quote, "Be polite, be professional, but always remember death."

Cops leave the safety of the police station and practice their critical thinking skills over and over, motivated by both efficiency and the desire to not get killed. Our internal harm might come from problematic adaptations of being a good cop. The following are four adaptations that stand out:

- Trusting less and controlling more;
- Being on guard for sudden violence;
- Police cynicism, skepticism, and suspicion;
- Separation from society.

Though necessary for self-preservation, these adaptations and adjustments can become over developed, out of balance, and misplaced. I did a lot of teaching before I became a cop, and I had an expansive vocabulary. But after a few years of patrol work and getting very good at talking with troublemakers for a living, I experienced a shrinking of my vocabulary and a narrowing of some of my views. Turns out that telling someone to "sit the fuck down" has a few applications in police work and almost none outside of police work. Being a cops' cop comes at a cost.

Along with EMTs, paramedics, firefighters and others, we are exposed to psychological trauma, the sights and sounds of the suffering of others, but what makes police work standout among other public safety jobs are these problematic adaptations. In this regard, police officers probably have more in common with corrections officers than they do any other public safety group.

Trust and Control

All police officers have had the experience of a complete stranger putting their trust in them, asking the officer to tell them what to do, to guide them through a fog, to give them hope. I was once taking a woman to jail and she whispered, "Officer, will you pray for me?" This is an intimacy of sorts, with the poor, the disenfranchised, the frightened, that cops know well. Years ago, I stood face-to-face with a man standing on the outside of a bridge railing; he threatened to jump to his death if we got too close. It occurred to me that in reality, there was nothing I could say or do to keep this man from jumping. So, without the illusion of control, a peacefulness, a clarity of mind came over me. And while we talked, there was a moment, I believe, that I witnessed the myth of isolation leave him.

Understanding cops has a lot to do with trust, control and stranger danger. We are often not *first responders,* but *last* responders, called when others or institutions have failed. Society asks officers to approach or confront strangers on its behalf. This is what patrol officers do for a living. Many of these strangers are not society's success stories; some are remarkably violent and lack impulse control, some have damaged brains. What these strangers hide in their pockets, their waistband, their mind, is unknown to the officer. What will happen when an officer walks up to a stranger? He does not know. How does he advantage himself? He does so by trusting less and controlling more.

Trusting less and controlling more becomes an absolutely necessary element of survival. In police work, where sometimes up is down and down is up, officers take control where they can, *and then some,* just to gain even the smallest advantage. And it only takes one near miss, to then fully commit to this kind of thinking.

The things we learn to survive, whether it is physical or social, become very well developed and protected. Although supremely useful in police work, trusting less and controlling more can have serious negative consequences in our personal lives. I first heard this concept described by Kent Williams, now a retired police chief, who speaks to police agencies under the business name Breach Point Consulting. Trusting less and controlling more can be our street mantra but applying it to our coworkers and our loved ones is destructive and interferes with healthy relationships.[2] Trusting less and controlling more does not work at home, households need a partner or spouse, children need a parent. If they need a cop, they can do what everyone else does — call one.

For the officer, a lack of control, a weakness or vulnerability, showing fear feels intolerable. On the street, it will be seized upon by those who would do us harm. Socially, because police work is tribal, a weakness might rightfully threaten the group. It is wise to be cautious about exposing our underbelly, but we must also know that the job has taught us some things that can both help us and hurt us. There is such a thing as too much of a good thing.

The event on the bridge ended like we would hope, but in a surprising way, not a grabbing on, but a letting go. He called me weeks later and left me a voicemail thanking me for being a friend. Whoever wrote the Serenity Prayer likely had been on one side or the other of a bridge railing. Asking for help, putting your faith in another, is a very human thing, a sacred thing.

Sudden Violence

Police work both requires vigilance and can cause hypervigilance. Hypervigilance is an "enhanced state of sensory sensitivity accompanied by an exaggerated intensity of behaviors whose purpose is to detect threats."[3] There are lots of dangerous occupations, some of which tally more physical injuries or deaths than police work. But in police work, we carry the extra burden of knowing that the source for most of our external physical harm comes from another human, someone wants us dead.

On guard for sudden violence, whether on the street or sitting in a restaurant, requires the evaluation of everyone as a threat or non-threat. Let us just say that a cop only needs to deploy that vigilance, act as a warrior, fight or stand ready to fight, less than 5% of the time. What percent of the time does she need to project that readiness? I do not have a number, but it is a lot more than 5%, possibly all the while she is in uniform and outside the protection of the police station. And because we do not lose our "cop-eyes" while off-duty, we may also have pangs of vigilance in our time away from work.

Cynicism

Police cynicism is an evolving pessimistic and suspicious outlook on the part of police officers toward their job, the public and society as a whole.[4]

I once heard a cop describe cops as being institutionalized, and patrol work as doing hard time.

In police work, the big eye-opener is seeing up close what people can do to each other. I remember standing with a senior officer at a bloody assault and hearing him muttering under his breath, "They're so violent. They're so violent." Pessimism and suspicion is only a natural consequence. I had a cop ask me when I was just months on the job, "Do you hate people yet?" I did not, and still do not. Although I can completely understand and relate to the feelings of disgust and despair from repeatedly witnessing stupid hurtful behavior which can translate into "I hate people." But I recognize that amongst cops, cynicism can come off as a well-earned clever grasp on reality. It can reach toxic levels where the less cynical are labeled naive, and unfit for *real* police work. Cynicism could be a coping mechanism for intense feelings we may not know how to handle, and it is not the duty of angry, crabby cops to ruin the "good old days" that new cops are in the midst of having. They should consider what I once heard a Minneapolis cop say, "Cops think the public doesn't know what reality is, but I'm not so sure we do either."

Cops do society's dirty work, dealing primarily with those who do wrong, or have been wronged, or are witnesses to the wrong. Cops' physical and mental survival requires adaptation. The learned response to the flash-bang of danger or the slow-burn of a steady diet of victim and victimizer, intimate exposure to psychological traumas and the suffering of others can look like the following:

- Pessimism

- Caring less and emotional numbing

- Physical exhaustion

- Misplaced application of distrust and control at home and elsewhere.

Cynicism, dark humor, and expecting the worst must have some important function or it would not be so common amongst officers. Expecting bad things can be useful, and cops do not want to die with their pistol still in its holster and a friendly grin or look of surprise on their face. Building trust with police officers includes not trying to talk them out of the things they need to survive. They do not need the extra burden of thinking that something unnatural is happening to them. Though certainly problematic at times, these responses are predictable and possibly necessary adjustments cops make for mental, emotional, and physical survival.

Cops have a job where we are lied to daily, and we are highly suspect of anyone that is not a cop, or is a cop that is a rank above us, or below us, or not on our shift, or works out of another precinct, or who seems to follow the rules too closely, or has never been in trouble, or who we do not have something to hold against them. Untrustworthiness can be deadly to the group, and those found out are alienated at best. In times of war, and other situations I am sure, those found to be untrustworthy, spies or traitors for example, were destroyed, and sometimes their families were tortured just to drive home the point. Non-cops might view our secrecy, distrust of outsiders, and how quickly we close ranks as all signs of dishonesty, yet often, it is a natural and reasonable form of self-preservation, a way to keep the organism alive and well.

Yet, despite all this, I will admit that I remain a little taken aback by how enduring the distrust of officers can be when I am trying to offer help; however, I understand it and do not fight cops too vigorously on it. I never *ask* people to trust me, nor do I try to talk cops out of their distrust or caution. A big part of helping others is getting past their resistance. The best way I know how to do this is to acknowledge their reality, their experience. In ambulance work, I would apply this to helping sick or injured children, a child struck by a car for example. The child would be lying in the roadway surrounded by cops and firefighters eagerly trying to calm his fears, and I suspect their own as well. They would gather around the child saying, "Don't be scared!" "You'll be alright!" The child, presumably believing he was not all right, and held down by strangers, screamed hysterically. I would arrive, calm my face, and look the kid in the eyes and say, "You look really scared! Are you scared?" He would scream, "Yes," and I would have his full attention, as if I was the only one who spoke English. My primary objective is not to deny officers' reality but gain trust by speaking their language and demonstrating trustworthiness.

Estrangement From Society

In my current EAP job, some cops come to me troubled by their own rage and anger. It might be unavoidable if you are paying attention, and just as valid an emotion as any. But as my wife pointed out when our kids were little, and they started hitting each other, "What is underneath the anger?" Usually it was a hurt feeling, sadness. Many cops start out like Boy Scouts and Girl Scouts, loyal, helpful, and kind. They try to make the world a better place, a fairer place. My observation is that cops have a lot of heart, and the bigger the heart, the bigger the heartache. Police officers do police work, meaning these mostly virtuous men and women do street-level work dealing often with not so virtuous, selfish and uncivil people. Cops clean up after other peoples' violence and neglect.

Many police officers love the work, in part because it is so interesting and enlivening, but what many additionally experience is estrangement from society. Some have been cops so long that police work is all they know. One cop told me, "I always assumed that people hated me and wanted to hurt me." Maybe some cops like it that way. Another cop told me regarding all the emphasis on "regaining" the public's trust, "I just want to go back to the days were most people just feared us a little." Neither view sounds like how society would consciously design police work, but it can be the outcome of doing the work that needs to be done.

Of all the side-effects of being a police officer, this estrangement can be the greatest burden and most deeply hurtful. Maybe some of my colleagues do not feel it or even care, maybe some prefer it. But it seems like a big price to pay for doing what society asks them to do, being the first to be called when people are frightened and the last to be called when all else fails. We literally help people sleep peacefully in their beds at night.

In this regard, cops can get lost in what started out as an effort to do good, to be good. I want to relieve cops of some of their sorrow, the stress of negativity, the fear that something unnatural has happened and that they have failed or are defective. All this painful heartache may exist for a good reason. Cops are willing to face bad odds; they just want to know what they are dealing with.

Cops Are Tough

Cops are tough. We are part of the working class who labor outdoors where we endure temperature extremes while wearing a uniform with body armor and a duty belt. Many of us have been physically injured, and we each have a vast mental library full of painful images and sounds. Surviving on our wits, we are mostly glad to do the work. None of us were drafted — we volunteered for this work.

Problematic Strength and Self-reliance

We may be better equipped to be a helper than to accept or seek help for ourselves. When I worked as a paramedic I found it nearly impossible to get an injured cop or firefighter to lie on a stretcher. As irritating as that was, I admired it, they were unwilling to be "cared for," with the public and their coworkers watching. We still got them to the hospital, but sometimes they insisted on limping in. Some of the macho tough guy and gal stuff is not all bad. Self-reliance, not indulging our weaknesses, manning up and the female equivalent makes us strong, and this can free us to help others or even ourselves in overcoming problems. This is fine to a point, as long as we recognize that our strengths can be our weakness, our weakness our strength.

We might become so accustomed to unease that we think we are supposed to suffer more than necessary, and we are good at hiding it. Or we do not fully realize we are in diminished health because of a slow decline. Chronic exposure to danger and discomfort can mute our alarm systems, and we wait for our problems to get really bad before something forces us to seek help. Even then, we may act only enough to turn the pain volume down a notch or two. There are times while talking with an officer that I know I am bringing him some relief, but I worry that my efforts make it easier for him to put off getting more help. A crisis can be a powerful motivator for needed change, but even a perfectly good crisis can be squandered. Wishing things would be different is not good enough. Within ourselves, we should be suspicious of any willingness to stop short of real substantial change in behavior.

Readiness for a change can come down to a couple of formulas: The pain of not changing is greater than the pain of staying the same, and the longer something goes untreated, the harder it is to treat. Waiting too long can be a damn shame because you lose time when you could have felt better, and you harm relationships. Some have said about necessary change, the hard part is deciding, the rest is persistence.

Special and Not So Special

In a crowd or a gathering of some kind, a police officer, even when off-duty, will react differently to a startling sound, a loud crash, a hostile argument, a bang or a boom. They will first look in the direction of the threatening sound to locate it, and then they decide if they need to attack it. While others cower or stand motionless with a hand covering their mouth, cops act; they identify threats and decide what to do about it. This is what makes them spectacularly different from other people. They may not have been necessarily created differently, but more likely, they had the right aptitude or interest, and they learned the skills, trained the brain and body, and accepted the responsibility.

Routinely, police work is all about trouble, trying to find it and being on guard in case it finds you. Walking alone in a dark alley or breeching a door goes against many instincts. And if another cop desperately needs you, you will do anything to get to him. There is a pride in knowing that you do a job that few can. Having a sense that you would sacrifice your safety for another requires some pride. And the practice fits better into a worldview if you are a part of a group that shares the belief. Many police officers love the work and may not view it as a sacrifice, but as already described, many experience an estrangement from society. The sheepdog makes both the wolf and sheep uncomfortable. Cops are parental in society. There was a time when cops were sometimes called "uncle," enforcing rules, often to those who have been poorly parented themselves; while as some eagerly point out, they also hypocritically break some rules at the same time.

Whether they feel special because of pride or estrangement, that specialness can be problematic. Embracing too tightly our separateness may be part of the problem when it comes to seeking good help. The cop's *I'm Special* list can look like this:

- We can't be understood *(which can feel true)*;

- We need special treatment *(which would be nice, but may not be good for us)*;

- Professional psychological help is especially risky for us *(which is not as risky as not getting help)*.

Bad Good Reasons

Cops can be very attached to their distrust of the administration or anyone outside the tribe. They will sight their *I'm Special* list as good reasons to not seek expert help and thus continue harmful behavior. But both a rational and an emotional argument can be made to the contrary. From a practical point of view, all cops have health insurance, and professional help may only be a phone call away. Emotionally, people are more alike than they are different. There is likely no better feeling than sharing one's fears and some secrets with trusted others and have it result in understanding and acceptance.

Sometimes the help we seek is just a new point of view, the fix can be as simple as seeing our situation or circumstances differently. A vague sense of unease is a nudge to do something different; a crisis is a two-handed shove. Being angry and bitter, for example, might be a reasonable response to the sights and sounds of police work, but staying in a prolonged state of anger could mean we are stuck and in need of further processing or re-orientation. None of this is without risk and asking for help can initially feel unnatural. Yet the impulse to tell another or ask for help is probably a very natural human impulse, just one that we as cops have developed strong control over. Officers need to be reminded that asking for help is part of an instinct to save themselves by way of saving their marriage, their valued relationships, their health and happiness.

If I imagine myself as a regular cop again, not the EAP director, I am not sure I would know when to ask for help. Is a low mood or lack of energy a normal temporary adaptation, or is it an early sign of trouble? I am not sure I know what the answer is, but the things that should get our concerned attention are a lessening or lack of interest in the people and things that previously gave us joy, an increase in anger, drinking too much, or a desire to isolate.

Adapt Some More

Police work can be more than just survival. We can thrive in this most noble profession. We owe it to those that have gone before us and to those who will follow. We must adapt and adapt some more; the alternative can be a slow stubborn death.

If cynicism is a natural consequence of police work, an inevitable survival tool for many, we can work to advance towards a new thought, a new point of view. We must continue to adapt. Whether we suffer from low-back pain or a low mood, the most disheartening thing is believing the condition is our new reality and that it will last forever. There are a number of things we can do to remedy a cynical mindset, some of which require lifestyle changes that are overdue anyway. Hope comes in the realization that people naturally move towards healing, can change their mind, have a mindset that is not set. We can work towards making negativity more productive, less destructive.

We struggle dutifully with trust and control between the worlds we travel as cops. We want to be safe, but we cannot armor ourselves enough. We need good weaponry as well, including the alertness and agility that comes with continued adaptation and being healthy.

Origins of Our Pain

The true origins of our pain may be unknown and undiscoverable as we sometimes recreate our history, remembering things not quite as they actually were. We may have felt a pain or a sadness and assigned the cause to an easy target, made a misdiagnosis. With this in mind, it may be worthwhile to consider that the origins of our mental and emotional distress may fit into one of two categories: police work or other causes unrelated to the job, such as what we were born with or the family we were born into. These concepts could be organized this way:

Police work:
    Hypervigilance
    Neglect or inattention to our health and wellbeing
    Instant Identity
    Spectacular Distractions
    Prolonged cynicism and societal estrangement

Born with or into:
    Nature, organic, biologic
    Nurture, childhood harm

Police Work

I once felt compelled to apologize to my barber for complaining too bitterly about something in the news, he replied, "That's okay, I think you know too much." The side effects of the police experience, or knowing too much, can be hypervigilance, cynicism and societal estrangement, which I spoke of earlier. Right or wrong, this can feel like something that *happens to us*. Neglect and inattention to our health and wellbeing is something *we do to ourselves*.

Neglect or Inattention Cops judge each other most on their vigilance; all else is subservient to alertness to danger. Given this mindset and the added daily potential for excitement, certain other less exciting, less immediate, more ordinary but necessary things can go without the care and attention they need. Just being a police officer gives someone a readymade identity; which we can put on, literally and figuratively, like a uniform. The problem with an instant identity, especially one as big and powerful as that of a police officer, is that we may not know how to handle it, thus the term "badge heavy." Additionally, a readymade identity could subvert the development of an identity independent of "police officer". An identity and interests beyond police work expands your world. When work is not going well, and you have a well-developed non-cop identity, it seems to have less impact, because being a cop is only part of who you are, not *all* of who you are. The less you want from the job, the less it "owns" you, meaning the less control it has over your happiness.

Police work is full of spectacular distractions, taking precedence over pedestrian things like adequate sleep, nutrition, tedious household chores, relationship responsibilities and family duties. When I started working as a cop, they joked it was a job where you got to fight, drive fast and talk dirty.

There can be lots of novelty in patrol work, the more intense, the more alive someone can feel. Like a drug, we can build up a tolerance and need a higher and higher dose to get the same effect. While we chase that "high," we may neglect more mundane things that keep us balanced and healthy. In time, after ignoring things in our personal lives, there may be a predictable crisis. When that crisis comes, we may say it is due to seeing too much death and destruction, where instead it was actually the result of personal neglect. Or the personal neglect made the death and destruction, inherent to the job, less manageable.

A cop once described to me the same sentiment this way: What if on your first day on the job you were given a new, or slightly used, squad car and told that it would be your only one for your entire career. How would you treat that squad? Here is the big difference; there is wear and tear from normal service, which can include all kinds of damage. Then there is excessive wear, off-road excursions (such as any number of vices), and poor maintenance. We should not lump them together as a common cause or expect anyone to feel sorry for us when our squad car will not drive straight.

Nature and Nurture

Our distress may not be directly related to police work at all. Often, as I have seen in others and myself, we have a tendency to find easy targets for our distress, such as blaming it on our work. For cops, much of our distress may be the result of growing pains. It is a job in which people often start young and stay a full career, thus we become full grown men and women on the job, as well as committed partners, husbands, wives, fathers, mothers, subordinates, and bosses. All of these life changes bring necessary stresses and responsibilities of their own.

Another possibility is that our distress may have a biological origin, such as a medical condition or diagnosable disease or disorder. Or it can be a result of our upbringing in the form of adverse childhood experiences. Often when I see cops in distress, I suspect it has more to do with what they brought with them to the job, than what the job does to them.

Reality of Our Situation

Where does our suffering come from? The big and little traumas of police work or the neglect of our own health and wellbeing? Maybe our adverse childhood experiences drew some of us to this work in the first place. It could be all of these, or none of them, it can be hard to know and it may not be knowable. What is possible, is to face the reality of our situation and get past the unhappiness blame. This is where we have a bad feeling, look around for its source and pick the easy target, our imperfect job, our imperfect loved ones and so on. Usually, we look for something outside ourselves. I have seen cops do versions of this, and I have done it myself — eagerly blaming others as if they conspired to limit my success. Or when a cop works too much and is surprised when it causes disorder in their lives or their marriage fails. What we need is self-reflection, basic skills, and the willingness to deal with the reality of our situation.

Look Within

Some things can be ignored, some things definitely should not be. We have to figure out which is which. What we cannot do is act like a victim. As police officers, we must be willing to recognize in ourselves what we often disparage in others, that is when able-bodied people are not self-reliant and claim victim status. Identifying as a victim can be like kryptonite and zap our strength. Rarely do you hear those who thrive under hardship speak at length about it. This is not the same as saying we can successfully ignore or outrun our past. I have driven many miles with a siren going, "on the whistle" as we used to call it. If you go fast enough you can out drive it, actually making the siren ineffective, as it does not project far enough ahead to do any good. Driving faster than the warning is very dangerous. We might live with the belief that if we can stay in constant motion, just keep moving, keep ourselves distracted, we can outrun the whistle.

What we should be motivated by, is our desire to not prolong suffering, to recognize a personal problem, and to take the necessary action to improve ourselves and avoid harming our loved ones. This requires something we are fully capable of, to look within and take responsibility for our own happiness.

Self-Awareness and Uncomfortable Emotions

It would be wrong, irresponsible and maybe even abusive to try to talk cops into feeling bad, or feeling anything in particular for that matter, when they do not. I know plenty of cops who carefully choose to not feel too much at work, but when their dog dies, oh boy, they look very human and fully functional to me. Instead of trying to adapt to some outsider view of what a cop should be, the cop should get to know himself or herself and learn to watch for signs of trouble, which could involve a failure to manage their thoughts and emotions or unprocessed psychological trauma.

Unease, an uncomfortable feeling, a nagging thought that something is not right, maybe even some anxiety and depression, may be our friend.

A sign of health and a wisdom telling us a change is needed or a change is coming. A recognition that what used to work in our life, no longer does. Our only real choice may be whether or not we become our true self, our authentic self, and that can take a lifetime. We might wrongly identify the bad feeling as the problem, rather than uncovering the true problem, that is, the act of trying not to feel it.

Progress comes with advancing our self-awareness. Fundamentally this means working from the inside out in order to feel better, by learning to both observe your own thinking and to feel your feelings. *What* you are thinking becomes less important than learning to observe the thought. With practice, you recognize that you are the "thought creator," and that emotions can be an indicator of the quality of those thoughts. Steven Hayes, a professor of psychology at the University of Nevada at Reno describes it this way, "Feeling your feelings, especially the uncomfortable emotions, even if only to pause and acknowledge them, is central to experiencing happiness and growth. 'Your ability to tolerate uncomfortable emotions is probably the broadest single psychological concept we know how to change, and with the biggest impact.'"[5]

Designed for Life

There is a price to pay for all of the direct experience of being a cop. Cops struggle mightily with trust and control, we must be on guard for sudden violence, we acquire cynicism, and we become estranged from society. These are necessities on the street when confronting strangers, picking up after other peoples' violence and neglect, and being parental to the weak, frightened or uncivil.

The things we do to survive, the things that come with being a really good cop, can have usefulness beyond the street and into the rest of our lives, but these skills can be overused — too much of a good thing. These adaptations can be like mirror-muscles that get overdeveloped or like the strings of a puppet that jerk us around. Once we have mastered the skills for our own street survival, the challenge is to move on to a more "full body" workout and take hold of the strings. By seeing our reactions and impulses for what they are and being more selective about what skills we use and when we use them, we control the strings rather than let them control us. We turn our problematic adaptations back towards the center.

We are designed for life, well equipped to navigate tough times, even benefit from them. We naturally move towards health and wellbeing. However, for whatever reason, we sometimes get stuck. Even then, without help we would probably eventually figure it out, but that could take considerable time, as in years and years and years. So, getting expert help can mean speeding up the process, minimizing the harm to our relationships and limiting the time lost before we feel better. The distress signals are designed to get your attention. They are your trusted partner. Part of maturing as a police officer and fundamental to officer wellness, is to turn back toward center and rebalance our power and might.

CHAPTER 2

STRESS, MOOD, AND THOUGHT

Get a New Thought

Stress, Mood and Thought Are All Connected

The police academy was tough, and it included ground fighting and exchanging knee and elbow strikes with academy mates half my age. I liked fighting and did well, but still ended up with a broken rib and a broken toe, both of which I kept hidden for fear of being kicked out or told to return for a later academy. This was my one chance at becoming a cop. The bone of the big toe was fractured down the center lengthwise, as I learned months later when I finally went to the doctor after graduation, and it never healed correctly because I had secretly casted it myself, hidden within my shoe.

To this day it will not bend. When I think of that toe, I feel a little pang of anxiety that I associate with the stress of the police academy so many years earlier. And if I really indulge my thinking, I might find myself remembering the humiliation of dropping out in the first round of a fourth-grade spelling bee, or other psychological traumas stored somewhere in-between the top of the head and the big toe, or between kindergarten and yesterday. The brain and the big toe are seamlessly connected, and our life history is as well.

What is the order of things? A low mood giving way to anxious thoughts, and then comes a throbbing big toe? Or, do the anxious thoughts arrive first, followed next by a throbbing toe, and then a low mood? Or can a low mood start with a sore big toe? The point is, as we know, the mind and the body are connected. Our thoughts and our emotions pull and push each other. And when it comes to psychological trauma, as Bessel van der Kolk says, "The body keeps the score."[1]

Just Because You Think It, Doesn't Make It Real

The connection between thinking and stress becomes clearer when we recognize that the feelings we associate with stress can immediately disappear with a new thought. Another perspective is that we can feel non-specific anxiety and quickly attribute it to an easy target, instead of just feeling it without being overly eager to label it or assign a cause regardless of accuracy. Perception is not reality, as people like to say. Instead, reality is reality and perception is just our best guess at it. Either way, we can be misled. Imagine if you went into your garage or a shed to retrieve something and in the dim light you were confronted by a snake, coiled up and ready to strike! You leapt back to safety, panting and heart pounding. In full light and full brain, you reconsider what you may have seen. That snake was awfully green and lying right where you keep your garden hose. In fact, you return to find that was the case, yet you fully experienced a near miss with a snake, as if it were real. Our beliefs, even our experiences may not be a reflection of reality. Just because you think it, or experience it, does not make it real. In other words, even things that do not exist can cause distress.

Our experience of stress is both learned and depends on our internals and externals. Internals include how our brain and body are wired, and our self-perception, which is made most evident in the things we say to ourselves. Our experience of stress also has to do with our externals, our environment, our relationship with others, our job, and our daily travels. Stress both keeps us alive and can kill us. With a deeper understanding of it, we can decide which.

Stress

Fishbowl

Stress, anxiety and worry are not the same thing but are closely linked. If our head were a fishbowl, these three could be different species of fish swimming around together, some we have fed more than others. Stress is largely the physical response of the body. Anxiety is more of an emotional response, often unconscious. Worry is a type of thinking and an attempt to solve problems.[2] Grouped together, they are mental or emotional strain, such as tension from overwhelming demands or even boredom. Rarely have I heard a cop say that they felt worried or anxious; once I heard a cop say he felt sad, but I think he was joking. Most commonly they lump feelings of mental, emotional and physical distress under the category of stress, and complain about feeling stressed out.

Each of these fish has different characteristics, but what they have in common is the fishbowl, or how we view or think about them. Ultimately you want to befriend stress and become the master of your thoughts, not a servant to them. This requires that you recognize how mental and emotional distress is not exclusively a mysterious force outside of us, but dwells mostly in our minds.

Just the subject of stress itself can be stressful, even the sight of the word "stress" is unpleasant, and "stress management" can feel like trying to fight stress with more stress. Most stress is not a result of what happens to us, but more a result of how we think about it. As a thought discipline, I avoid talking directly about stress and prefer instead the subject of healthy thinking. Humans are designed to think of the worst possible thing when they are stressed and that process can make the situation more stressful, so stress management can involve interrupting our thinking or reconsidering how we label things. We might be more relaxed and grateful if we reframe how we describe things. For example, experiment with describing your own life, or an otherwise challenging situation, as a happy or grateful person would. One cop describes going home as leaving work chaos for the happy chaos at home. This reframing was played out in a flash once for me while camping with one of my sons and his Boy Scout troop. The tents were old military style, made of canvas and placed on pallet-like decks. Some tents were in a shady breezy location while others were in the swampy, densely-wooded and mosquito-infested area. We were assigned to the more Amazonian spot, as I was gathering up my grievances in my head, my boy blurted out, "Boy, did we luck out!"

Because we can change the way we respond, get a new thought, I find it more accurate and useful to frame any lesson about stress around self-awareness, thinking habits, practices that maintain an orderly life, and getting adequate rest.

It Is Good to Have One In a Crowd

Although excessive worry and anxiety may be habitual and self-perpetuating, some freedom from the burden can be achieved by knowing that some people are setup this way and the rest of the group benefits. Humans and advanced animals can vary amongst themselves considerably on how much stress they experience. Some creatures have greater sensitivity to certain stressors than others, and this can be very useful to the group. I once read a study that described how within a group of herd animals a small percentage will be more sensitive to stimuli. These extra-sensitive antelopes, for example, can be seen looking around frequently while the others graze. The rest of the group depends on them to register the approach of a predator and set off a stampede. The herd could not survive without them. There are humans with this *special* skill.

Stress Inoculation

I recently met a man who upon learning that I was a police officer told me that he had done a ride-along with his son, who was a police officer. Although I would guess that the son tried to show his father an exciting time, it was likely a relatively ordinary tour of duty. Yet, the father described the experience as being extremely stressful, and stated he had not yet fully recovered from it even weeks later.

In a typical day, week, or year, a police officer might experience more uniquely stressful events than some people do in a lifetime, and some cops like it that way. While developing a health and wellness survey of officers, I had to change the phrasing about stress from "Do you experience stress?" to "Do you experience *extreme* stress?" Most surveys do not ask things like: Have you argued with someone today? Taken someone into custody who did not wish to be taken into custody? Have you done CPR on someone while loved ones stood by weeping? An ordinary stress exposure assessment will put a police officer off the chart compared to many.

The alarm system built into us to fend off danger can go on and off in seconds, such as when you evaluate the body language of an approaching stranger, or it can be continuous as you fret about your finances, marriage or kid troubles. Like noise pollution, an alarm that stays on all the time can begin to be ignored.

How do cops and others survive stressful work year after year? Some do not and are dying a slow death, but most do fine by adapting and learning when and where to turn their stress responses on and off as needed. We get good at stress. In police work, responding to emergencies may not be the job's biggest stress factor, but it can be used to illustrate stress inoculation, where a few big dramatic events or numerous smaller repeated exposures can teach us how to lessen the impact of future exposures. It is exciting to work in a job where you are beckoned into action by a cry for help or the voice of a dispatcher. A job where you look for trouble and your "office" is a vehicle with emergency lights and siren. Thankfully, when we repeat the experience enough times, most or all of the excitement wears off, ideally, our alertness remains. There are enough false alarms in emergency services work that eventually you learn to underreact, to avoid the rollercoaster ride. Repeatedly, a "baby not breathing" call turns out to be a relatively benign febrile seizure, a "man walking down the street with a rifle" turns out to be a teenager with a toy, fifty people fighting in the street turns out to be two fighting and 48 watching. Saying to yourself, "I'll believe it when I see it," might be smarter and more self-protective than cynical.

Repeated exposures to events build experience. We learn how our mind works, body reacts, and how situations unfold. Things essentially become more predictable, and we welcome the occasional novel event because it is enlivening. Ideally, we do not figuratively fall asleep on the job, but stay somewhat relaxed while still alert, ready to act when the bell rings or the suspect's behavior changes. You know when a cop is reading the landscape and does not like what she sees, catches a whiff of trouble, has her game face on, gets in the zone. When it is "go-time," she values a little stress for peak performance.

The flip side of this is being too relaxed. I noticed that when I worked with a regular partner, who was also a friend from the academy, I felt lulled into a stupor as we laughed and talked the whole shift, interestingly, I also sometimes felt more vulnerable, and counterintuitively, I felt safer working alone. A friend of mind was working with his good buddy and they arrived on an alarm call, only to hold open the door for the burglar who was carrying out a TV. Being completely relaxed can make for a dull-minded cop. The Yerkes-Dodson law tells us that we perform best at a sweet spot between too little and too much arousal or stress. The law dictates that performance increases with physiological or mental arousal, but only up to a point. When levels of arousal become too high, performance decreases.[3]

Stress Is Bad If You Think It Is Bad

We can build resilience through both lifestyle choices and changing how we think about things. It is wrong minded to try to eliminate stress. Even if it was desirable, it is impossible, being without stress would be like being without bones. Rather, we can think differently about stress, create a stress narrative that helps us see stress as our friend. Kelly McGonigal, a health psychologist and the author of, *The Upside of Stress — Why Stress Is Good for You, and How to Get Good at It*,[4] describes how a "meaningful life is a stressful life" and that changing your mind about stress can change your body's response to stress. She cites a 2012 study lead by Abiola Keller which demonstrated that the deadliest stress comes from the combination of lots of stress and the belief that stress is harmful. Individuals experiencing lots of stress while accepting, utilizing and embracing stress as their friend enjoyed better health and survival outcomes than even those with less stress.[5] The physical stress response can be viewed as positive, preparing you for the best performance. The goal should not be to get rid of stress, but to get better at stress, see it as helpful and as a means to create the "biology of courage."[6]

Many cops are well practiced in managing stress out on the mean streets. This stress can arrive suddenly, like an alarm. We associate patrol work stress with specific situations, like chasing after bad guys. Through prior experience, practice or visualization we advantage ourselves. Often the threat is clear, and we know what our response should be. Usually within 30 minutes or less, we get the "all clear" signal, and we return to our on-duty baseline.

Patrol work stress can feel good and act as an escape from the stress that really gets you down, the stress from inside the police station, what we like to call "politics," or boredom, or from the stresses at home, the grown-up demands of a relationship, raising children, paying bills, and maturing. These forms of stress can be numerous and vague, without clear boundaries, solutions or a timeline. The cop must transition between these different worlds daily, unlike soldiers for example, who might spend long periods in the battle zone and long periods away. In a twenty-four-hour cycle, the police officer navigates both police vigilance and a personal life. As a comparison, what if soldiers were in the battle zone for eight, ten, twelve hours, then were magically transported home and ate dinner with the family, helped the kids with homework, slept in their own bed. And instead, what if a group of patrol cops were deployed to the streets for months at a time, taking turns keeping watch as they slept in abandoned garages. The point is, cops and soldiers have some things in common, and although the analogy is incomplete, you can imagine that in some ways, being in a battle zone for extended periods could in some ways be easier than what officers do by switching in-and-out of the work stress on a daily basis for years and years. The police guardian's greatest challenge becomes the transition, taking off the armor and returning home as spouse, partner, parent, son, daughter, neighbor and friend.

Too Much Stress Is a Lack of Recovery

We may agree that we can think differently about stress, anxiety and worry, and we may have some success viewing it as our friend. But even a friend can get on your nerves, demand too much of your time, or wreck your stuff. Too much stress can start to feel less like bending and more like breaking, putting us into a kind of survival mode where we think primarily in terms of worst-case scenarios. As stress signals overload our body and mind, we may lose some rationality making even smart people do dumb things.

If we ignore the warnings long enough, our body will finally refuse to play along and lets us know. According to Dr. Martin Rossman, "The body will stay tense all day long if it keeps getting alarm signals from the brain, but if you take the time to send it 'all clear' signals once in a while, the body will relax, it will let go of stress physiology and go into a relaxed state, where it repairs, refreshes and renews itself. It will also learn different ways to react to stress if you show it how, with this, you get back in control of your brain instead of letting it run away with you."[7] Unmanaged, stress is both unpleasant in the here and now and the biggest factor in accelerating aging.[8]

Often, we do not know what is enough until we know what is too much. Too much sun is a sunburn, and another stress event without recovery can be like burning a sunburn. We can all handle a lot more adversity than we may think if we can build up our reserve or find some recovery. Experiencing feelings of being compromised, overwhelmed or hopeless does not mean we are broken, instead, it means we have not recovered. Returning to a baseline of wellbeing is ideal, a temporary recharging will do. If our baseline health is good, all of this is more easily attained.

In his book, *The Worry Solution: Using Your Healing Mind to Turn Stress and Anxiety into Better Health and Happiness*, Rossman describes how most of the things we worry about never come true. But because we think that our worry kept them from happening, our brain gets a little reward and we develop a worry habit. He contends that the goal is not to eliminate all worry; there is a lot to worry about, and it is a survival skill that serves us well. Instead, we can benefit from breaking the unconscious bad habit of worry, by managing our thoughts and learning how and when to worry more deliberately.

Dr. Rossman advises sorting our worries by good and bad. Good worries are the worries that you could possibly do something about. These are worries that help you avoid danger, solve problems, or find opportunities. With some thoughtful consideration, imagination and by accessing your own wisdom, our natural and sometimes surprisingly clever problem-solving abilities can be encouraged. Rossman describes bad worries as those that you cannot possibly do anything tangible about, no matter how badly you want to. These may be worthy things to be concerned about, but if you keep going over them, you will make yourself stressed, depressed and anxious. You need to conserve your energy for the things you can do something about and use your mind for good.[9]

Recovery and Stress Management Techniques

In my parents' time, stress management was known as relaxation, and some methods were remarkably simple. For my mother I think it was a hot bath, my father, cleaning the garage. But life seems more complex now and so are the remedies. Either way, this is what we seek, the feeling after laughing with friends or getting lost in play, the physical sensations of shoulders down, easy full breathing, and a relaxed face.

Up North, as we say here in Minnesota, I once saw a sign that read "Do nothing right." If we read it the way I think the author intended, it suggests a skill and purpose in doing nothing or doing less. When you are out putzing in the garage and you wife calls out, "What are you doing?" And you answer, "Nothing," you are not trying to deceive her, but you are doing nothing in a way that is productive. It is hard or maybe impossible to literally do nothing. Instead, putzing in the garage, or power washing the driveway or cooking is relaxing because you are engaged in a simple activity that takes your attention away from yourself or thinking too much.

Cops have described to me feeling stress return as they prepare for work after days off. They might treat this as evidence that something is wrong with them or their job. That may, or may not be so, but I encourage them to recognize that the ability to identify the onset of stress, and maybe going so far as to know where it first appears in their body, is progress.

It is important to believe that you can manage your stress, and that depends on healthy routines and intentional behavior. These healthful routines can be purposefully inserted throughout your workday, rather than exclusively compartmentalizing rest and recovery for after work. The whole 24-hours of each day is your life, not just the small segments you claim for yourself. You can improve your baseline of health and dull the sharp edges of the potentially harmful things in your life. Practices such as conscious breathing, yoga, meditation, mindfulness, and healthy thinking can make you both more mentally flexible *and* sturdy. There is nothing new here. These are ancient practices, make them your own.

Conscious Breathing. Conscious breathing is pausing to focus on your breath. It can be as simple as just noticing your breathing and taking a slow, full deep breath. It may be helpful to visualize expanding your torso upward and diaphragm downward, while also expanding your ribs horizontally.

You may already be practicing conscious breathing if you are a hunter or mastered this at the gun range. "Proper breathing techniques are important for any shooter, not just those who hunt. You won't be as accurate as you can be if you don't breathe properly. And you definitely won't overcome buck fever if you're breathing irregularly and uncontrollably when a buck steps out. Make a conscious effort to inhale deeply and exhale slowly. Continue this process over and over from the time you see the deer, until just prior to the shot. This will help your muscles to relax and brain to focus."[10]

Yoga. The term yoga means union. Some might extend that to mean union of mind and body where you harmonize thoughts and actions. For some, yoga is a philosophy of life and includes many different types of yoga, but in the Western world we usually think of Hatha yoga. This is a group of postures, breathing techniques and meditation. Some benefits of yoga can be decreased stress, lower blood pressure, and better sleeping. It is easy to find a yoga class and excellent videos on the Internet.

Meditation. The author of *10% Happier,* describes meditation as "simple, secular, scientifically validated exercise for your brain". Three steps of meditation are: 1) sit with your back straight and eyes closed; 2) notice the feeling of your breath coming in and your breath going out, focus your full attention on this feeling; 3) Notice when your mind wanders and start over, start over, and start over as needed. It is an exercise, try-fail-start again. You are breaking the habit of constant projection and rumination by bringing your focus into the now.[11] For more on meditation see Chapter 11.

Mindfulness. Mindfulness is a centering technique that, like meditation, involves being more aware of the present moment. It is the "ability to know what's happening in your head at any given moment without getting carried away by it."[12] It is not uncommon to have a thought or experience and immediately respond with a feeling such as anger, with little to no buffer between the prompt and the reaction. Mindfulness is the practice of noticing your thoughts and reactions and learning to respond more wisely, rather than just reflexively.[13]

Healthy Thinking. Healthy thinking is not just positive thinking; it is a deliberate process to retrain your brain that starts with raising awareness about negative thoughts, learning new skills, practicing and creating new thinking habits. A healthy thinking practice begins with noticing in yourself how common our negative self-talk is, then replacing it with what is literally or factually true. Asking others and yourself, "How true is that?" is fundamental to a reality-based life. Healthy thinking will be explained in full later in this chapter.

Stress and some discomfort are part of a meaningful life. If your work lacks meaning for you, I suggest you go looking for it. Because police work, possibly all work involves some suffering, and without meaning, it is all suffering. The goal is to view stress differently and to our advantage while learning to avoid unnecessary stress.

Mood

Emotions

Cops readily recognize the value of a gut feeling, and they are well practiced in managing their own fear in face of danger. Police work exposes you to the raw emotions of others, and in order to function on the job, you purposefully suppress your own emotions in response, for good reason. The job is full of despair, and if you had to constantly feel what others were feeling, the work would be impossible. The goal is not free expression of our emotions at work, which would not be in anyone's best interest.

As a cop, you are rightly encouraged to suppress emotions and demonstrate control over them. Many cops have learned this the hard way regarding expressing anger on the job, "If it feels good – don't do it or don't say it." Managing your emotions also serves as a tactical advantage and lets your coworkers know they can rely on you to stay focused on the task. But as a human, experiencing emotions are as fundamental to survival, growth and development as good nutrition and exercise. Their presence, and the importance of feelings, can be hard to grasp because they take the shape of a wave rather than a solid object. Emotions can be elusive and often we are so unpracticed at acknowledging them, that they are hard to identify or correctly name. They may get mislabeled or incorrectly assigned to the wrong source. Emotions may get stuck inside or find their way out in less healthy ways.

Raw emotions, like fear from danger or grief from sudden loss, might be more manageable because they may be more obvious, tangible, and visceral. It is the subtle emotions like sadness and shame, which might scare cops the most and sneak past their defenses. They include feeling heartsick with disappointment about the job, feeling isolated among your coworkers, or feeling abandoned by the community you thought you were protecting. If you really want to frighten one of these brave men and women, and most people in our society, then ask them to sit quietly alone in a room with their thoughts and feelings. Maybe your biggest deep dark fear is that your emotions will overtake you, if so, know that the best way to manage your emotions is to be aware of them. Be reassured that even the most intense or unpleasant emotions last only so long if just given their say. Normally, when emotions are felt they kind of pass through us.

It is not hard to convince cops they should pay attention to the importance of emotions. Kevin Gilmartin has sold lots and lots of books with the words *emotion* and *law enforcement* in the same title. Had he not included the word survival, we may have never picked it up. I have heard *Emotional Survival for Law Enforcement*, quoted or referenced by cops more than any other document, including the Constitution or Bill of Rights.

My observation of my father's generation was that men exercised fewer options to express emotion. Their emotional energy tended to be channeled into emotions such as excitement or anger. I credit my father with great emotional progress, he was expressive and openly affectionate to my mother and us children, even though his own father had modeled stoicism. I was rather comfortable with a range of emotion and modeled that for my boys, yet I did not disregard the stoicism either, in fact I am grateful for my ability to also contain some emotions.

The stoic cop, man or women, is neither good or bad, not better or worse than those who are more expressive. For all cops, mental and emotional progress is becoming more emotionally aware. A starting point can be noticing your emotional triggers, for example, the feelings that accompany boredom or the things that get you angry. The next step would be to explore what is below the anger or what you might be trying to *not* feel when bored.

We *can* have it both ways, a healthy emotional life where we recognize our feelings and express them in the settings of our choosing, and at the same time manage and control our emotions on the job and elsewhere. This can be achieved by practicing acknowledging emotions and managing your thinking. The intent is to develop greater competence with emotions as a way to expand our life skills, not make us soft, more vulnerable, tamed or in need of fixing, but instead more conscious.

Cry to Expel

The strategy of identifying and experiencing feelings might need to be relearned because somewhere along the line, it became necessary to forget what you already knew as a child, to cry or act upset when you felt really sad, hurt or afraid. Adults do not necessarily need to cry to be emotionally healthy. But some feelings and strong reactions cannot be easily reasoned away. Crying, for example, can be reflexive, like a startled reaction is reflexive. It is often a quick way to feel better.

Your own discomfort with someone else's crying, especially another cop, can result in trying to alter their behavior or rush in with a bunch of platitudes to make you feel better. Fortunately, I am not uncomfortable when someone else cries, which I believe gives them a lot of space. However, I know of no one who likes crying at work, so my first priority would be to give them privacy from others if needed. If they say, "Sorry, I don't know what's wrong with me." I might say, "What makes you think something is wrong with you? Take your time." And if I can tell they are fighting back tears, I do what I would hope someone would do for me, I help them breathe through it. Just advising them to take a big breath will sometimes let it pass. I do not encourage or discourage a cop from crying but recognize the immediate psychological and physiological benefits from this very natural process.

Some things in police work are very painful and trying to suppress strong feelings can actually make things worse and last longer. I work with a cop whose father was also an officer. As a child, he remembers a time after his father shot and killed a bad guy, and the father cried for two days. My friend and his brother (also a cop) viewed their father as strong and mighty, but one who also cried. *(Story retold with officer's permission.)*

Emotions Must Have Their Say

It seems that emotions must have their say, at least internally. Trying to control our feelings has utility, but once we achieve a certain proficiency at it, we may do well to loosen our grip on the controls and allow more free expression in the right time and place for our own good. Trying to control feelings can just make them stronger. I saw a parallel to this in patrol work when dealing with an excited or angry victim or witness. Not giving them their say only made them more insistent. And if I was momentarily too busy to listen because a scene was too hectic for example, I found nothing more calming than to look them in the eye and say, "I want to hear what you have to say, but let me get this crowd settled down first."

A nagging feeling, unease, mental discomfort all exist for a reason, to get our attention, like an infant's cry, to get us to attend to something important. While there are plenty of people that could benefit from turning down the emotion and turning up the rational thought, we as cops, could benefit from learning to feel the feeling, let it have its say, and then move on.

When I started ambulance work just out of high school, I wanted to be as hard and tough as the guys I worked with. And in the early stages of my career I seemed to achieve that. But then it started to worry me; suppressing emotions became too generalized, where I did not seem to feel anything, neither good nor bad, just numb. I looked around, expanded my view beyond those that seemed to hold a tight fist around emotions and realized, there were some ambulance workers that seemed more able and willing to feel bad about bad things. I continue to recognize the need and still honor a young paramedic or cop's need to learn to hold it in. But career progress means further evolution and a deepening relationship with sad or bad feelings.

This can be illustrated by what I hear in my EAP job from older and more senior officers following a bad call at work, like the homicide of an innocent or dealing with all the raw emotions of a victim's family members. The older cops say, "You gotta check on the young cops, that was a really bad one." Yet, I have observed that the young cops seem less affected and they shrug it off. I suspect because they have no shelf to put the new experience on, maybe they do not know where to file it. It is just a new experience, one among many, and they may not be able to put it in perspective. It is the older cops that seem to be the ones that really need attention, who suffer more. They are the ones that immediately know which crowded shelf to put the screams of the mother on, which over-stuffed file to place the image of the dead child. I suspect, as I know in myself, the older cops seem to have softer hearts. They do not want any more suffering, and they know what matters most in life.

Even if we acknowledge logically, that feeling our emotions is good for us, it is natural to want to avoid discomfort, and some emotions can be extremely uncomfortable. I have had moments when I was so eager to distract myself from an unpleasant thought, that, while driving, I have reached down to turn on the radio only to realize it was already on. Distracting ourselves from our own thoughts and feelings does not mean we are damaged people, but rather we are in need of relearning how to feel our feelings. Effectively dealing with strong feelings, can be as simple, yet challenging, as letting them have their say. As Steven Hayes, a psychology professor points out, "People's willingness to sit with uncomfortable emotions and find some meaning in them — feeling, learning, moving on — predicts positive outcomes in their ability to lose weight, quit smoking, stick to an exercise program, learn new software, do well at work, and survive burnout. And it correlates with all these other things like reducing depression and anxiety."[14]

Important Pause

Feeling feelings is not the same as being more emotional. Instead it can be viewed as an important skill that requires practice. There is a benefit in just pausing and acknowledging a disquieting thought or an uncomfortable emotion. Take for example, you get home from work and the first thing you want to do is have a drink, or after days off you start thinking about going to back to work and you have a strong urge to play video games for hours. Having a drink or playing video games is not necessarily bad, however drinking to relax or playing to distract could be. When you find yourself doing something in order to feel different, the first step is to pause and take notice of it, not to deny yourself, but just stop and acknowledge that you might be trying to avoid an uncomfortable thought or emotion. Next take a deep breath and quiet yourself. Then identify the feeling if that helps. Follow this with feeling the feeling without judging it or trying to talk yourself out of it. Maybe it is a feeling of anxiety, or fear, or anger. Underneath that, maybe sadness or shame, or maybe if you are really skilled, you can just feel it without naming it. Taking a brief pause can do wonders, and then have your drink or obsessively play video games if you still want to, or perhaps you no longer need to and go on to something else. It can be transformative to insert a layer of self-reflection between the uncomfortable emotion and the action intended to avoid feeling it. The pause is a great first step and may well be enough to change your relationship with your inner self as you seek progress, not perfection.

> **Important Pause:**
> 1. Notice it
> 2. Ask yourself, "What am I feeling?" or "What am I trying to avoid feeling?"
> 3. Feel it/sit with it momentarily
> 4. Proceed

Timed Pause

Some uncomfortable thoughts or feelings invite themselves in and refuse to leave demanding more time than you want to give them. Another practice can be to limit uncomfortable thoughts and feelings that are intrusive or seem insatiable. Instead of trying to block them out, which likely will not work and in fact may intensify them, set a time limit. For example, "I'll think about this or that intensely for exactly four minutes and then stop." You may find that you can only worry intensely for so long and it is the act of fighting it, trying not to feel it, which makes it worse.

A Deep Good Feeling

With time and practice, acknowledging your feelings and feeling your feelings will become more natural. You may learn to further differentiate between a shallow good feeling that comes from gossiping, assigning blame, or relieving a craving, and the deeper good feeling that comes with connecting with your more authentic self. This could be compared to the difference between fast food and a home-cooked meal. We can use a deep good feeling as a guide to wellbeing. Self-exploration includes a willingness to examine what we attribute our "good" or "bad" feelings to.

Thought

The Boss

Once there was a man who went hours at a time without a conscious thought, and he was just fine. Both the unconscious and the conscious brain are exquisitely well designed for our survival. We have a little brain and a big brain, an old brain and a relatively new brain. The little or old brain is at the center in the area around the top of the spinal cord. We might think of it as our animal brain. Evolutionarily, the conscious mind, the bigger and newer brain, the part of us that knows we are us, the more "human" brain, that can think, feel, imagine, talk, and plan, grew out of the animal brain. This is why humans can play a piano and lizards cannot, besides the fact that lizards do not have the dexterity or the patience for piano lessons.

The term executive functions refers to the higher-level cognitive or thinking skills, used to control and coordinate thoughts and behaviors. "Who we are, how we organize our lives, how we plan, and how we then execute those plans is largely guided by our executive system."[15] The term is a business metaphor, the executive manages all major tasks of the company so it can operate most efficiently and effectively. The executive is the boss of the brain and does our best thinking. Executive coaches or sports psychologists work with clients to develop the boss. As children, our parents may have had this role, and in some ways, as young cops, our supervisor or senior officers may have, but as we grow and develop, we become more and more our own boss.

Dr. Martin Rossman describes the brain as "the central processing unit of the body. It receives data from the body as well as from its own emotional and memory centers. It assesses the situation, makes decisions, and sends out orders and messages to the body, most of this process is deeply unconscious, but it can be influenced by our conscious mind." The body has an intelligence of its own, but does not filter the signals and sends them off without prejudice. It is a good soldier and "always tries to do what the brain asks it to do, it cannot always do it, but it tries."[16]

We do not have to live with whatever drops into our head, we can learn to manage our thinking moment-to-moment to our best advantage and learn which alarms to pay attention to. This includes getting a new thought or choosing one thought over another. We can ask more of the executive, and that executive is us.

Changing Your Mind for Good

By learning to observe your own thinking, you can in effect add a layer of thought between one thought and the otherwise automatic next one. Take charge of your thinking.

Consider this, it is possible the vast majority of the thoughts we have today are the same thoughts we had yesterday, and the same from last week and maybe a year ago. New thoughts are relatively uncommon. And if you do not seek them out, they are probably rare. Maybe this is why a crisis can be so impactful; we get forced out of an old way of thinking. A crisis is squandered if it does not result in thinking in new ways. This may also be why curiosity or a new experience can be so enlivening.

Thoughts exist without words I suppose, but the only way I know how to examine a thought is to investigate, as best I can, the words attached to them. What we say to ourselves matters. Our big life plans and our moment-to-moment choices are guided by this inner voice and unless we challenge ourselves, the vocabulary in that self-talk can remain small and negative.

The conscious mind lives essentially in the brain. We can change our minds, get new thoughts, think better, and practice healthy thinking. Healthy thinking includes the practice of blocking or quickly extinguishing negative thoughts; it is a deliberate process to retrain your brain that starts with raising awareness, learning new skills, practicing and creating new habits, or ways of acting. Many of us already have the habit of negative self-talk. Changing our mind for good becomes a matter of identifying common thoughts and reactions and loosening our attachment to them, allowing for a bit of healthy distrust of them. Some of our own thinking needs to be talked back to, some with a whisper, others a shout.

Wisdom comes from experimenting with both trusting your gut and doubting your thinking. A big learning curve for me starting out as a cop, and one that needed constant reminding, was to recognize the danger of thinking that others, namely criminals and ne'er-do-wells, thought like I did. As cops, we learn to think in ways that are on the one hand very useful and on the other hand unlike most of society. In fact, increasingly, we share in common with criminals that we both think like criminals, and we play cat and mouse trying to predict each other's next move. Necessarily, this means suspecting more people of sinister intent, and sometimes reacting or acting aggressively when they do not immediately cooperate or follow commands.

In police work, we sometimes admire quick and decisive action, even if it is wrong. Although deliberate action can feel really good by relieving the stress of not acting, some distrust of our thinking, and the thinking of others can be helpful. Doubt can be extremely valuable and even life-saving because it allows an alternative way to see the world.[17]

A willingness to challenge your own thinking is a good start. At the most rudimentary level, it can sound like this, "I don't know, maybe I'm just being paranoid." Or feeling stressed and noticing the next thought is wanting to stop at the liquor store. Cops study human behavior for a living. We can benefit from studying our own, starting with observing our own thoughts as part of a lifelong journey of self-awareness.

Healthy Thinking — Steps to Changing Your Mind

Healthy thinking is being more realistic or accurate about your thinking. In many ways unhealthy thinking is really just mistaken thinking often expressed as negative thoughts. We were probably designed to ruminate on negative thoughts and emotions as a means to avoid the situation that led up to those negative thoughts and emotions. When you are stressed, tired, or otherwise out of orbit, you may reflexively revert to negative self-talk. This may have been adaptive and useful for survival, to think of the worst-case scenario when you feel compromised in some way. Although this may have its usefulness, it can be overdone, tiresome and unpleasant.

At the root of this unhealthy, unhelpful or mistaken thinking are cognitive distortions which are exaggerated or irrational thought patterns that are believed to perpetuate mental and emotional distress.[18] Psychiatrist Aaron T. Beck laid the groundwork for the study of these distortions, and his student David D. Burns continued research on the topic. In *The Feeling Good Handbook*, Burns describes how to challenge your own thinking and provides a list of what he describes as distorted thinking patterns, or what we might describe as negative thinking.[19]

Negative self-talk can take several forms, and our sometimes-lazy brain may have its favorite negative thoughts. Examples of negative self-talk are numerous and available lists are worth reviewing. They tend to follow common themes such as low self-regard, criticism and blame. Others include magnifying, exaggeration, overgeneralizing or sometimes the other extreme–minimizing.[20] We can recognize unhealthy thinking in others and ourselves when we hear phrases that include: categorizing situations as all-or-none, jumping to conclusions, responding with woulda-shoulda-coulda, and quickly labeling yourself or others ("I'm bad at this or that," "They think I'm stupid").

A shortcut to healthy thinking can be simply distracting yourself from a budding negative thought before it gets ahold of you. Replace it with a positive thought or rebuttal based on factual information or a kinder interpretation. An example could be your response to receiving an unsettling look from a coworker. Instead of getting carried away with a narrative that they are angry or disapproving of you for this or that reason, you simply say to yourself, "I'm not sure what that meant, if it meant anything at all, or maybe they are worried about something."

The strategies to overcome negative thinking habits and to incorporate healthy thinking habits require steady practice at first and then an occasional refresher. Once you begin, it is difficult to return to unhealthy ways of thinking because you now see the link between thought and emotion. Furthermore, you may recognize that with a low mood you have a tendency to interpret things negatively. As you interact with others you will be continuously reminded of your progress as you observe how they are sometimes misled by their negative thinking. Dr. Karen Lloyd first introduced me to the subject of healthy thinking and the steps to incorporate it into a new life routine. Lloyd is a national speaker on behavioral health topics and emotional resilience.

We can think of this process as "thinking about thinking" and reframing those thoughts. You start by recognizing that your thoughts and feelings are connected, and then observe your own thinking, taking note of any negative self-talk. Replace the negative self-talk with talk that is factual or literally true, fair and kind. Repeat this process until you form a new habit and healthy thinking becomes more natural to you. The result can be that you will think well and feel better. Below are the steps for healthy thinking:

Step 1: Observe your own thinking.

Step 2: Take note of your negative self-talk.

Step 3: Replace negative self-talk with talk that is factual or literally true, fair and kind.

Step 4: Repeat until you form a new habit and healthy thinking feels more natural.

Step 5: Think well and feel better.

Each step is described below in more detail:

Step 1: Observe your own thinking.

Begin to notice that you are actually quietly talking to yourself in your head. This is called self-talk and you do it all day long. Once you become aware of this, you can make observations of what you are saying to yourself.

Step 2: Take note of your negative self-talk.

If we were to keep a tally of our negative self-talk, our running commentary and pessimistic internal responses, we might be impressed by how often we frame our experiences and interactions negatively. It can go like this when getting on an airplane for example, "I hope the pilot isn't drunk. First class–those guys are lucky. My-god, can you not lift your own bag into the overhead compartment. Do you not know we are all waiting on you? The air will be bad in here. I see a baby, please don't let me sit near a crying baby." This can all take place in seconds and your face will take on a serious or crabby look while you project hostility, which is met with the same.

Step 3: Replace negative self-talk with talk that is factual or literally true, fair and kind. A void in information will always be filled, and rarely with something that is not salacious or dramatic. Facts are best, but not always available; fair and kind is a good substitute or placeholder. They are how you would want to be treated, how you would like your actions or intentions to be interpreted.

When you are in a low mood, what comes out of your mouth can be regrettable, and what you say to yourself suspect. If we wish to be the executives rather than servants of our brain, we must recognize that our first thoughts, designed for short-term survival, can be evaluated for their usefulness and subject to being replaced.

Step 4: Repeat until you form a new habit and healthy thinking feels natural. Just being aware of a negative-thought tendency in yourself and others can be all it takes to add a layer of healthy doubt about immediate thoughts. You can also apply the healthy thinking practice to any upsetting situation, your own or someone else's. This could be why when we feel upset, our impulse is to tell someone. The wise part of us may be seeking a different point of view or perspective.

Step: 5: Think well and feel better. The healthy thinking steps of raising awareness; learning new skills and practicing to create a good habit can be simplified as:

- Watch (observe what you or others say to themselves)

- Check (to see if it is literally true)

- Correct (substitute a true, fair and kind statement)

Dr. Lloyd suggests that to make this a lasting change, you actually keep count of the frequency of your negative thoughts for a few days. Then you continue noticing negative self-talk and start replacing it. You may even notice that you have favorite negative phrases. Dr. Lloyd suggests that after this process, healthy thinking changes can last for a year, and if you do a yearly refresher, the changes can become a permanent component of your wellness.[21]

By recognizing that your thoughts can mislead you, you can develop a healthy distrust of them, and also recognize that your mood can be an indication of the quality of your thoughts. With healthy thinking we improve our mood and enjoy the stability of dwelling in a more fact-based world. Getting a new thought can be likened to emerging from a cold, dark and damp basement to the sun-warmed kitchen of restoration. Once experienced, all other forms of thinking feel incomplete or undeveloped.

If you want to be a better partner, family member, friend, neighbor, cop, or whatever, start acting like one and stop letting your negative thinking jerk you around. By better managing your thinking, you can control your perceptions, direct your actions, and willingly accept what is outside your control. It is far better to manage your thoughts than to let reflexive thoughts manage you. Alternatively, you can let your actions influence your thoughts. For example, want to feel better, smile; feel powerful, stand up straight with shoulders back, fill your chest with air. In these cases, let your thoughts and feelings follow your body's lead.

CHAPTER 3

FITNESS, EXERCISE AND NUTRITION

Use It and Choose It

Sturdy Pioneers

Conscious efforts to be physically fit and eat well have become necessary in modern times, whereas in our great grandparents' time, it was likely part of daily life. I am embarrassed to say that my ninety-year-old father-in-law's big hands are stronger than mine. I have never known him to exercise per se, but he is active and lifts heavy things on his farm. As it turns out though, my hands are probably stronger than the college kid's down the road per the 2016 study of such things.[1] Each generation has its own challenges, and those who went before us proved, in many ways, to be sturdy people who routinely attended to healthy mental and physical routines out of necessity. We are fortunate in that we do not have to pull out our own aching tooth with pliers or live without heart surgery, but we do have to be more attentive and deliberate about making choices moment-to-moment in favor of fitness, exercise and nutrition.

Healthy thinking, healthy eating and being physically fit and active are all connected, and not overly complex; the difficulty may be in how ubiquitous the temptation is to do otherwise. It is more a matter of giving our health the time and attention it requires, and we should not rely solely on motivation. Feeling motived can be helpful to propel you into action; however, for many, the voice in your head saying 'just do it' more often says, 'I don't feel like it.' Even Olympic athletes in training combat a constant voice that says, "Stop, you had enough."

You want to be forever active and free of discomfort and disease, and this may still be possible even if you have been in a few too many squad car crashes. For some, this requires major changes, others, small adjustments, both require getting your mind right. The best thinking comes from a well-fed, well-rested and well-loved brain. The best eating requires planning and limiting unhealthy options, the best physical fitness is being active, and the best exercise is the one that you enjoy or will do. We achieve fitness success by being attentive moment-to-moment to healthy options, recognizing our ability to choose, stacking the deck in our favor by planning ahead, and relying more on reasonable routines than sometimes fickle motivation. The opposite of this is what an old Hennepin County paramedic once described as the ambulance drivers' motto, "Why stand when you could sit, why sit when you could lie down, if you see a donut, eat it." Cops survive by the motto, action beats reaction; well, a long-term survival motto could be action beats inaction. This action means attending to your overall physical fitness. We achieve this with exercise and good nutrition. This chapter focuses more on reminding you of fitness priorities and less on specific techniques. There is a wealth of information easily available to tailor to your own lifestyle, body type and personal preferences.

Exercise

"The best exercise is the one you'll do." — Officer Jim Class

Officers must see physical fitness as a lifelong pursuit requiring daily contribution. What is most important is showing up. A number of times I have had an unhappy cop tell me, "I gotta get back in the gym." Some of these people were in really rough mental and physical shape, and I know they were imagining working out like they used to, years ago with more available time and a younger body. I try to reframe that good, yet sometimes overly ambitious intention by encouraging them to design success, "How about starting with a daily brisk walk in your neighborhood."

I do not like to exercise, but despite this, when I became a cop, I dedicated myself to physical fitness with a focus on strength and endurance. My goals were hierarchical. First, do not embarrass myself in the academy. When I hit the street, it was three-fold: 1) reduce the risk of injury, 2) gain and maintain confidence in my physicality and thus officer presence, and 3) win the big fight. For me, the motivation to exercise was both survival and wellbeing, and I saw no other way to achieve that then to show up daily, make it part of a daily routine.

A lawful order is only as good as the ability to enforce it. I was an averaged-sized cop and had been in a fight or two before coming on the job. I started in the era of what we understood to be the ask-tell-make style of dealing with "No" people. "No" people being those that say or act out "no" to even the simplest of lawful requests. Officer directives most commonly started by asking, failing that, telling or commanding, and as a last resort, making or going "hands-on." Sometimes you progressed slowly, other times their behavior dictated skipping a step. Sometimes the spark that ignited my fierceness came without any forethought. I had seen more than once a bad guy looking into my eyes trying to judge my resolve, as I calculated my next move. Once, in the void between saying and doing, a bad guy and I stared at each other, I was deciding where best to hit him. Suddenly he smirked and stepped back as I had commanded him. I tell this story because my resolve, backed by my fitness, made it possible.

There was a time when police departments hired cops based on size, big men who did not need to learn a lot of fancy cop techniques. Their best defensive tactic was being physically decisive and letting a troublemaker know that the hand of a man was upon them. A strong back and a weak mind are insufficient for the complexities of modern policing which places more emphasis on brain than brawn. Today, cops come in all shapes and sizes. For all, fitness remains a critical aspect of the job.

Just as the pen in our pocket is the best route to justice, our persuasiveness and physicality, not the tools on our duty belt, are the best route to getting people to do what we need them to do and follow lawful orders. In conclusion, we must be physically fit to consistently do our best police work. The stress of the work, as well as aging in a physically demanding job, requires that we attend to physical fitness. The elements of fitness include strength, flexibility, mobility, endurance, injury prevention, and pain management.

Use It or Lose It

Gaining and maintaining strength, flexibility, mobility and endurance can occur by a variety of means. For the police officer, exercise has a role beyond just physical fitness which includes confidence and command presence. Police work is a physical job, so injury prevention and recovery, and sometimes pain management, is a goal. Information on exercise is readily available, and most cops know what they need. More useful is to avoid misinformation and fads, and instead focus on general principles.

The body has a "use it or lose" bias. If you do not use all our parts, you are sending the body the message that they are not needed. Stressing bones and lengthening muscles can be a way to send the body a different message.

You have certainly seen people who have given into physical decline, which compounds itself, their world seemingly becomes smaller and smaller. As a patrol officer, I was frequently amazed at the people I dealt with who were much younger than I but appeared and acted much older. Markers of good health and longevity in elderly people are things like balance, ability to get off the floor unaided, grip-strength, and unobserved walking speed.[2,3] Though you may not feel elderly yet, the things you are doing or not doing now will show up later.

Strength

One of the fundamental benefits of building or maintaining strength is looking better, but other benefits include improved vitality, confidence, posture, metabolism, and free and easy movement. For many cops, weight lifting builds size, camaraderie and can relieve stress. Big muscles can look good, and I understand why cops believe that big muscles equal strength and make you safer. But strength can also come with agility and functionality. Many cops have discovered that the big strong looking guy may not be able to use that strength in a functional way, and it is the "wiry" little guy that puts up the best fight. Additionally, cops can be hard on their own bodies as they seek to gain muscle by subjecting themselves to imbalances between push and pull muscles, joint strain, improper technique, or too much pounding. For them, I would add, try not to hurt yourself and know that if you choose strength over flexibility, you may actually be shortening your muscles and harming your joints.

Flexibility and Mobility

Fitness can correctly be judged by how well we move. What we notice about children and spry old people is how they move, or we might be shocked by how a relatively young person can act nearly disabled. Free and easy movement is a sign of health, and it may be the best defense against injury, giving us our greatest advantage when responding to resistance and aggression. Cops can get in the trap of thinking they only need strength and large muscles which can result in decreased flexibility. The best use of your whole musculoskeletal system is to have both strength and flexibility.

Endurance

When I was a paramedic in Minneapolis, we would on occasion respond to a call where the cops had been in some kind of brawl. I remember being impressed, and alarmed, at how gassed the strong and fit young cops could get. Cops know that a struggle lasting longer than a minute or two is unusual but can be extremely taxing. Sometimes we fight to win, sometimes winning is hanging on until help arrives. During the difficult part of my workout, when I want to stop, it helps to imagine I am in the fight of my life. In a sense, we are all in a fight for our lives, but now the fight is against becoming too sedentary, and thus signaling our body that we are ready to lie down and die.

Injury Prevention and Pain Management

We start out in life with full and easy range of motion, but due to overuse or injury, our ease of motion can decline. The loss of one area of full function naturally affects other areas. At the same time the body can adapt. For example, some with low back pain have perfectly fine-looking x-rays, while others with defects can be pain free. A few scars, both physical and mental, might be the cost of police work, but if we do not recover well, injury can diminish our quality of life.

The pain cycle is natural and predictable: back pain signals to us that we have injured or over-taxed the low back. Pain is an essential survival signal indicating there is a problem; maybe we need some rest and recovery, or to lose some weight. If discomfort continues, we cannot help ourselves, we avoid pain, which often means reduced use, which results in a weakening of muscles (atrophy), which result in more pain and so on. The bones, ligaments, tendons, discs, and muscles of the back are all living tissues that need oxygenated blood, improved blood flow comes through movement.

Low back pain is common for police officers. Apparently, the human lumbar spine has not fully evolved for walking around upright, and you are worse off if you wear a duty belt and sit in a squad car. For what we ask it to do, the spine should have been created bigger and stronger, and the discs around L4-L5 can be the weak spot.

Because the low back is inherently vulnerable, we must consider what we can do to minimize the reality of our anatomy and keep moving. It is vital that you do not abuse your lower back by using poor lifting technique, sitting too long, or neglecting to minimize the hazards of wearing a duty belt. Additionally, you should develop your core strength to support the low back.

Other areas of the body are also vulnerable based on design. The more versatile the joint is, such as the spine, shoulders and knees, the more vulnerable they are to injury, whether from high school sports or police work. These joints need time to recover from overuse or injury and should be protected. Protection comes from both strong and long muscles and improved flexibility.

Be Active

Sitting in a car or at a desk for long periods of time is very unnatural, but the more we do it, the more we may want to do it. A certain amount of restlessness is helpful, as it prompts you to get up and move. If it is true that robots are taking over and planning to kill us, they are doing it with escalators, TV remotes, and cell phones. At the very least we can outsmart the robots by operating our electric toothbrush with our reaction hand. The body can be thought of as a class of kindergarteners, they behave best after nap time, but are otherwise restless and want to run, jump, push, pedal and have fun. If the best exercise is the one that you will do, then the very best is the one you did not even realize you did.

Nutrition

Good nutrition requires planning, which requires forethought and time. When you were a baby, you were surrounded by mostly healthy options and quantities of food. You lived twenty-four hours a day with personal chefs and were completely dependent on them to make healthy choices for you.

Some people mature into healthy eating naturally and easily, for many however, it can be a colossal daily struggle. Besides requiring planning, healthy eating can be more difficult because eating can be social, emotional, and subject to a constant barrage of temptation. Grocery shopping and eating well require discipline. The list of challenges can be overwhelming, so a good start is to relieve yourself entirely of the concept of dieting. Weight loss should be a result, not the goal, of healthy eating. Know that when we focus on not doing, we can trigger a sense of deprivation. Instead we can focus on doing, by being more deliberate about what we eat, and more mindful when we eat. Focusing on dieting can fail. Success comes with an attitude and lifelong practice of doing things that are good for you.

In retrospect, there were times in ambulance work when we dutifully did procedures that were later determined to be harmful. I could write a chapter on nutrition, but before the book was published, some advice would become obsolete or wrong. Presently, our modern human diet does not resemble early man's pre-agricultural diet. Even if we wished to eat as we may have been designed to eat, those foods cannot be easily found. We are surrounded by food that a purist would not even recognize as food. With this in mind, saying less here is more, and maybe I should stop at, dark green is good, sugar bad. You will have to decide on your own what you want, how you are going to get it, and what you will have to sacrifice for it.

As with exercise, the nutrition changes you need to make may require only small adjustments or an overhaul to try to get off medications, reverse pre-diabetes, or remove impediments to fully participating in life.

Choose Food Carefully

When you were younger you could burn green wood in your fireplace, now you seem to require good dry logs. You need a steady and pleasing fire, not smoldering garbage or a raging bonfire. You can no longer just grab what is available; you have to spend some time and energy foraging. The foods most likely to be good for you are those closest to their natural state, or have no added ingredients, some describe them as foods that can be grown or killed. Bad foods are manufactured and have lots of added ingredients, in some cases, so many it might be better for you to eat the carton.

Consider What Food Means to You

As we struggle to make healthy food choices it might be good to know that we are fighting against more than convenience and cost, and for some, food and emotion can be closely linked. In lieu of deep psychological evaluation here, it may be useful to at least know this and be willing to acknowledge when you are eating emotionally. You can pause and ask yourself, "What am I feeling? *When Food Is Love* by Geneen Roth is a good book for further reading on emotional eating.

Plan Meals

Thoughtful meals start with meal planning. A useful step is to make a meal plan or menu for a week or even a month at a time. Shop from a list according to your menu. This seems like a lot of work, but with this in place, in the end you can save time, money and calories. Failing to plan will result in relying on inspiration, hunger cravings or emotion. Think about what meals you are going to have and gather only what you need for them. Do not bring problem foods into your home. And if you need snacks, think instead of them as small meals, which you also plan, such as packing a handful of nuts and carrots for the time you know you get hungry between breakfast and lunch.

A weekly meal plan can help you anticipate challenges, whether they are situational triggers, holidays, or shift work. Additionally, having a set breakfast and/or lunch, that you eat most days, that is healthy and something you enjoy or at least like, sets you up for eating healthy most days. This will also make it easier for you to always keep the ingredients you need on hand and help you feel grounded even during challenging times.

Learn what works best for your body and lifestyle. For some, a strict adherence to a meal schedule is needed, others can ignore the clock and successfully learn to eat when hungry and until full.

Thoughtful (Mindful) Eating

Rather than treating meals like an afterthought, inserted into a busy day like some task to fend off hunger, make meals a social or meditative process when possible, a time that you extend good care for yourself. Retrain your eating habits by practicing slowing down, careful chewing, setting down your utensil while chewing and feeling grateful. I grew up saying grace before eating. This act added a layer of thought and gratitude for the food and the event of eating.

The opposite of thoughtful eating is to grocery shop while hungry, deny ourselves and feel deprived, or eat emotionally without first at least pausing to check-in with our feelings. We need to listen to our body and learn to better attune ourselves to eat when our body tells us to eat, stop eating when full, and when eating, just eat.

Outwit Bad Food

"If I have just one, I won't be able to stop." Food scientists design manufactured foods that way, like chips, which do not grow on trees. I really like chips, but I do not like being manipulated. Some foods are specifically designed to activate certain taste buds and have a short-lived affect perfectly timed to the rhythm of reaching for another. So, when you indulge, outsmart them and their voodoo science, by taking the quantity that you plan to eat before the first bite. Whether it is chips, ice cream or candy, do not eat from the container. When it comes to sweets, a handful of nuts beforehand can fill you up and also slow the sugar blast.

Just because you can buy a pair of foam dice and hang them from your rear-view mirror does not make them legal, just because products use words like "low-fat," "whole grain," "organic" or even "healthy" does not mean they are good for you. The less manufactured the better.

Eat Mostly Healthy, Most of the Time

If you are a food purist and that works for you, great. If not, you can invent your own eating strategies, such as: eat healthy six of seven days, or eat healthy 80/20 or 90/10 percent of the time. Some people have success with incorporating fasting, as early humans were likely forced to do. An example is limiting eating to an eight-hour window, in effect fasting for sixteen hours between dinner and breakfast. I have found this 8/16 fasting routine remarkably easy to follow, helped in part because I only follow it strictly five of the seven days, which allows for social events that involve food. An added benefit is that I eat less and enjoy meals more. During the eight hours, I do not necessarily limit what I eat, but I find eating is guided more by hunger and stopping when full. I also find the fasting period eliminates grazing or snacking when bored.

If you have an occasion of eating poorly and feel bad about it, do not punish yourself. Instead do the next right thing and return to good. The other day a cop handed me a Dilly Bar. I am naturally thin, but struggle with too many sweets. As a child, we did not have many treats and I tend to hoard sweets or do not want to waste an opportunity to get something free. I was nearly finished before I thought to myself, "Yuck, that was too much." I could have said, "No thank you," or stopped before finishing. Instead of going down a tunnel of self-loathing, I thought to myself, "I'll do better next time."

You owe it to your fellow officers, your loved ones and most importantly yourself to make it a priority to attend to your fitness throughout your whole career. Information and advice about fitness is plentiful, and most officers have coworkers who are willing to share their expertise. Some larger agencies like mine have a full-time fitness coordinator, annual physical assessments and provide officers access to the gym while on-duty. But the one factor that remains in all of this, it's up to you to *use it and choose it*.

CHAPTER 4

SLEEP

"Let's Be Alert Out There"

Sleepy Cops

We need restorative sleep to be healthy and happy. Sleep deficiency is common among police officers[1], and the practice of working while sleep deprived is embedded in police culture. Good sleep hygiene requires discipline and is critical to officer safety and especially challenging for those who do shift work.

Good sleep hygiene, though difficult to achieve, might be one of the easiest things to identify as a worthy effort for wellness. There is no ambiguity about how much sleep is good or bad for you, and the risks of failure here are clear. "Fatigue is an identifiable risk. Let's take responsibility and manage that risk." says attorney Gordon Graham, a risk and liability specialist, retired California Highway Patrol captain and founder of Lexipole. In an interview with Force Science News, Graham indicated "fatigue played a significant role in at least 3 officer deaths that he's aware of in recent months, in just one state alone."[2]

"Administrators won't talk about it," Graham says, "but our cops are ticking time bombs for lack of sleep....If a big rig runs off the road, we take that driver's life apart for the previous few days, looking at his sleep log, among other things. But when something tragic happens with a cop, we don't analyze for fatigue." He continued, "Wouldn't it be interesting to know how many hours of sleep officers have had before some of the controversial shootings that have rocked law enforcement? Or to correlate citizen complaints with officer fatigue?"[3]

It is hard for many officers to get good sleep consistently. At my police department, about a third of the officers report six or less hours of sleep daily.[4] We treat sleep like something that can be negotiated down, expendable, a luxury rather than a necessity. "Humans are the only creature that deliberately deprives themselves of sleep."[5] Although we can occasionally get by on less as an exception, we routinely need good sleep day after day. Unlike the ability to store calories in the form of fat, humans have not evolved any way to "store" sleep. We can skip meals, and in some cases be better off for it, but not so with sleep, yet we act as if we can.

We need 7–9 hours of sleep every day. More than that is not necessarily better, and if you think less than 6 is adequate you are wrong and fooling yourself. "If we could have done away with any of this, Mother Nature would have a long time ago, 3.6 million years have put this in place".[6] On less than seven hours sleep, you will have measurable impairments.

Imagine a world where everyone had a naptime — cops, robbers, everyone. Or maybe just the good guys could take a nap, which would save lives and be a huge crime fighting advantage. Historically sleeping on the job was rightly seen as a dereliction of duty. However, some agencies have implemented a systematic process for taking a nap on duty, and I believe sleep experts would support this.[7] But this is largely an adaptation to odd work hours. The best long-term approach is to deal effectively with sleep problems and to adapt or legislate good sleep practices or sleep hygiene.

I worked with cops who routinely got off work at 2 AM, drove home for a few hours of sleep and got up with the kids, maybe took a nap later and then came back to work. I knew one cop who during the day slept on the floor, lying across the top of the stairs like a human baby gate. I have worked every hour of the day or night, and even worked 24-hour-shifts as a private ambulance paramedic. I also crashed an ambulance on my 25th hour with one-hour sleep. By the time I was a cop, my kids were mostly grown, and I was able to go to work each day well-rested and well-fed. It made all the difference in my performance and enjoyment of the job and in my family life.

We know we are making progress when cops no longer boast of the lack of sleep as a sign of toughness or dedication, competing on who can suffer the most, and instead, treat sleepless pride like someone boasting about not brushing their teeth or changing their underwear. We should expect people to come to work well-rested, the work requires it, and the public and coworkers depend on it.

Stupid Pill

The reason we sleep is much more than just fending off sleepiness or exhaustion. A lot goes on while you sleep, including processes that "reenergize the body's cells, clearing waste from the brain, and support learning and memory. It even plays vital roles in regulating mood, appetite and libido."[8] It would be accurate to envision our brain as being slightly damaged doing all the tasks needed during wakefulness and viewing sleep as a time to repair that damage. "Although a sleeping person may appear inactive, some functions of the brain and body are actually more active during sleep than when we're awake."[9] Without enough sleep all of this maintenance work goes undone and we will not think, feel or act normal.

While we have been dozing, David Grossman, psychologist and author of *On Killing and On Combat*, has been saying that we have been acting stupid, the reason, a lack of sleep. According to Grossman, sleep deprivation is a reason officers commit suicide, make ethical mistakes, and use excessive force. If you want to 'fix' the police, he thinks federal regulations should require police officers have the appropriate hours of sleep before they are allowed to patrol. "You see a video of a cop doing something stupid? I'll bet you anything that the cop was sleep deprived. Sleep deprived people do stupid stuff." He calls sleep deprivation the stupid pill.[10]

No one cares more for the wellbeing of cops than this man, and this is what he tells everyone. If cops were required to test alertness prior to going on duty or throughout the tour, we might be shocked by the results. The lack of corrective action is likely due to one, underestimating the extent of the problem, and two, the enormous cost of correcting it. Yet we are already paying dearly for our lack of adequate sleep.

There is a strong connection between sleep deficiencies and the negative effect on mood and mental health. Additionally, prolonged sleep deprivation can put cops at a significant increased risk for suicide.

The list of harmful effects of sleep loss is exhausting. A lack of adequate sleep, less than the necessary seven or eight hours, impacts how we think and act, and how well we live. "In the short term, a lack of adequate sleep can affect judgment, mood, ability to learn and retain information, and may increase the risk of serious accidents and injury. In the long term, chronic sleep deprivation may lead to a host of health problems including obesity, diabetes, cardiovascular disease, and even early mortality."[11] More succinctly, a lack of sleep ages you, it shortens your life.

In a radio interview, professor Mathew Walker and author of *Why We Sleep*, explains that all the major diseases killing us in the developed world have "significant and many of them a causal link to lack of sleep. If your goal is to have a life that is free of disease for as long as possible, then increasing sleep amount is going to be essential. We also know that from large scale epidemiologic studies a very simple truth: the shorter your sleep, the shorter your life." He adds that the advice that you can sleep when you are dead is mortally unwise and if you adopt that mindset, "Your life will be shorter, and the quality of that now shorter life will be significantly worse."[12] Of all the risks inherent in police work, a lack of sleep would be a dumb way to die.

How We Think

The cops we think of as just lazy may instead have been made dumb by poor sleep hygiene. People who are sleep deficient have impaired cognitive abilities. Psychologists and sleep researchers have pointed out that "Sleep deprivation impairs attention and working memory, but it also affects others functions, such as long-term memory and decision-making. Partial sleep deprivation is found to influence attention, especially vigilance."[13]

Furthermore, sleep loss impairs judgment. What should be frightening to cops is that it makes their own assessment of alertness unreliable. Expert Phil Gehrman has said that, "Sleep-deprived people seem to be especially prone to poor judgment when it comes to assessing what lack of sleep is doing to them." If you think you are doing fine on less sleep, you are probably wrong because you are asking the wrong person. For a cop, dozing off at the "office" could mean crashing into a parked car or much worse. "Studies show that over time, people who are getting six hours of sleep, instead of seven or eight, begin to feel that they've adapted to that sleep deprivation –they've gotten used to it," Gehrman says. "But if you look at how they actually do on tests of mental alertness and performance, they continue to go downhill. So, there's a point in sleep deprivation when we lose touch with how impaired we are."[14] Getting by with a lack of sleep is, in reality, becoming accustomed to feeling crappy most of the time.

In a discussion with two sleep experts and educators from St. Thomas University, I described my belief that I had been able to snap out of a stupor to rise to the occasion. They looked at each other and smirked, kind of like two cops do when the sloppy drunk says he just had two beers. At first, I was annoyed, but upon reflection felt embarrassed that I had been delusional and they knew better. I had been the classic public safety worker, thinking I had superpowers and could routinely power through disadvantages. And because I had done it before without obvious bad outcomes, I thought I could rely on it. As I have heard others say, the problem with luck is that it runs out, and relying on luck in police work is dangerous. People who think they can routinely get by on 6 hours of sleep are doing just that, getting by.

How We Act

Physically, the importance of sleep can be illustrated with a comparison to working out. Not only is 8 hours needed for recovery after working out, but less recovery time negatively impacts performance, gains,[15] and can lead to more injuries.[16] If you have to choose between extra needed sleep and time in the gym, choose sleep.

Sleepiness cannot be controlled. When we reach our physiologic limit we will fall asleep, even while driving. Falling asleep or poor performance may not be our biggest concern, but it should be because a lack of sleep will affect our performance and may lead to big mistakes.

Making Mistakes. In police work, moment to moment our judgment is tested, and in a flash, so can our critical thinking skills. Big mistakes can cost lives; and little mistakes can rapidly become big mistakes. "Insufficient sleep may not have led the news in reporting on serious accidents in recent decades. However, that doesn't mean fatigue and inattention due to sleep loss didn't play a role in these disasters. For example, investigators have ruled that sleep deprivation was a significant factor in the 1979 nuclear accident at Three Mile Island, as well as the 1986 nuclear meltdown at Chernobyl."[17,18] Investigations into the grounding of the Exxon Valdez oil tanker, as well as the explosion of the space shuttle Challenger, have concluded that sleep deprivation played a critical role in these accidents. In both cases, those in charge of the operations and required to make critical decisions were operating under extreme sleep deprivation.[19,20] Same old story, big mistakes on little sleep. We each have our own examples and collections of near miss stories, they do not rise to the level of Chernobyl, but they could have cost someone their life or livelihood.

Dr. Rajaratnam and his colleagues studied the impact of insufficient sleep on police officers and reported, "although in-the-line-of-duty death rates in police have decreased by almost half since 1972, the proportion of deaths due to unintentional injury have shown little change and in 2003 were greater than the rate of felonious deaths. Across 2009-2010, more than one-third of in-the-line-of-duty deaths were due to motor vehicle crashes. Driver sleepiness is a major cause of motor vehicle crashes, and excessively sleepy individuals have an increased risk of having more crashes and more serious crashes. Obstructive sleep apnea exposes individuals to increased sleepiness and a 2- to 3-fold higher risk of motor vehicle crashes. We found that excessive sleepiness is common in police officers, with almost half reporting having fallen asleep while driving and about one-quarter reporting that this occurs 1 to 2 times per month. This is despite police officers apparently recognizing the dangers associated with drowsy driving; in a survey of North American police officers, almost 90% regarded drowsy driving to be as dangerous as drunk driving."[21]

When your body and mind sense trouble, you might not identify the cause as a lack of sleep, you just know something is off. A reasonable survival mechanism could be to react as if everything is a threat and maybe overreact to perceived threats or catastrophize things. Sleep deprivation can make us more volatile. Rajaratnam also studied the effects of sleep disorders on police officers and one conclusion was that "(t)here may be a biological basis to our finding that those who screened positive for a sleep disorder were significantly more likely to report displaying uncontrolled anger toward a citizen or suspect." He cited the research of Yoo Seung-Schik whose brain imaging studies found "that those in a sleep deprived state were unable to appropriately govern behavioral responses to negative emotional stimuli."[22]

Sleep Problems

Chronic inadequate or non-restorative sleep can be due to one or more of the following: poor habits, a less than ideal sleep environment, competing or conflicting life priorities, or a diagnosable sleep problem such as obstructive sleep apnea, insomnia, and shift work sleep disorder. There are others, but these are the big ones for cops.

A study of thousands of cops showed that over 40 percent screened positive for at least one sleep disorder, the majority being sleep apnea, with one-third of officers screening positive.[23]

Sleep apnea is a condition where a person's breathing is interrupted during sleep. People with this disorder stop breathing many times during the night and can wake up feeling tired. **Insomnia** includes having trouble falling asleep or waking up and not being able to fall back asleep. Insomnia can be caused by disruption in circadian rhythm, psychological issues such as anxiety or depression, or medical conditions. **Shift work sleep disorder** occurs when you have sleep difficulties because of your work schedule. Basically, you have a conflict between your circadian rhythm and your work schedule. Symptoms are insomnia and excessive daytime sleepiness.[24]

The majority of people with sleep disorders are undiagnosed and untreated.[25,26] This is unfortunate because very effective treatments exist, and untreated sleep disorders can lead to all kinds of diseases, weight gain, mental disorders, and diminished quality of life. Sometimes the solution may be as simple as a change in either routine or the sleep environment. If problems persist, you should consider consulting with a sleep specialist.[27] Perhaps the first place to start would be visiting web sites such as the Harvard's School of Medicine, Healthy Sleep website for all variety of tips and ideas for better sleep.

Alcohol. A survey of police officers revealed that ten percent of respondents frequently or very frequently used alcohol or other substances to aid in sleep.[28] Although drinking alcohol may help people fall asleep, it negatively impacts REM, or dream sleep, and effectively harms sleep quality.[29]

Sleep Medication. It is critically important for the officer who is getting little to no sleep to seek professional help. Doctor prescribed sleep medications can be useful in helping some people sleep better, but pills should not be seen as a long-term solution for better sleep. Doctors rarely prescribe them for more than three to four weeks. Sleep medications can become less effective when used for a long period of time and also have negative side effects. There is no ideal long-term sleep medication.

Healthy Sleep Fundamentals

With good sleep our memory is better, our skin is better, and our mood is better. In addition, our ability to fend off, or recover from illness, injury and psychological trauma is improved.[30,31] Good sleep requires discipline, a conscious effort to make it a priority, and a commitment to good habits and routines. If this sounds too intense and contrary to drifting off to sleep, consider creating your own bedtime ritual and treat yourself like a child; parents know that a bedtime routine such as a gradual calming down, a bath and story time can make all the difference.

Basics of Good Sleep:

- **Make sleep a priority.**

- **Maintain a regular sleep schedule** by going to bed at the same time, but more importantly get up at the same time, every day. When you wake, seek sunlight.

- **Establish a bedtime routine** that is gradually calming while avoiding bright lights or stimulation.

- **Create the best sleep environment** by keeping the bedroom dark, cool, quiet and reserved mostly for just sleeping.

- **Avoid alcohol, caffeine and large meals close to bedtime.**

- **Exercise regularly,** but not too close to bedtime.

What to Try While Lying Awake

In order to train your brain to associate the bed and the bedroom with sleep, you should avoid staying awake in bed for long periods. Sometimes as we lie awake, especially in the small hours of the night, life's big questions and big fears can occupy your thoughts. Or your mind races with to-do lists or concerns. The next morning neither may seem so important or frightening. It can help to write down lists and concerns, so you do not need to keep them active in your head. Relaxation methods, such as Dr. Andrew Weil's 4-7-8 breathing technique listed below, may also help you fall asleep.

1. Exhale completely through your mouth, making a whoosh sound.

2. Close your mouth and inhale quietly through your nose to a mental count of four.

3. Hold your breath for a count of seven.

4. Exhale completely through your mouth, making a whoosh sound to a count of eight. This is one breath.

5. Now inhale again and repeat the cycle three more times for a total of four breaths.[32]

If you have not fallen back to sleep after a few minutes, consider getting out of bed and doing some light yoga or stretching, or read a book under low light.

Good Sleep

A healthy night sleep begins with you starting to feel sleepy as the evening progresses. Doctors Michael Howell and Brent Nelson provide the following description for good sleep. "You should fall asleep within 10–15 minutes. You should not have to force yourself to feel sleepy, just like you do not force yourself to feel hungry. It is normal to wake up occasionally throughout the night, sleep is not one homogenous state of unconsciousness, normally we wake every 1½ hours [often without realizing it], then fall asleep again in 5–10 minutes. When you wake in the morning you should not be able to sleep later. Short-term sleep deprivation can be made up, chronic can't. You should be able to catch up on all the extra sleep with as little as 2 hours of extra sleep on the days off."[33] Naps should be between 20–30 minutes max, and at least six hours before bedtime.

Odd Hours — Shift work

Shift work has some advantages, but in regard to sleep it can be problematic, especially for the overnight shift. A 2016 report titled, Shift Work and Sleep Quality Among Urban Police Officers: The BCOPS Study, revealed that, "the overall prevalence of poor sleep quality was 54%; 44% for day, 60% for afternoon, and 69% for night shift."[34]

Shift workers tend to be continually sleep deprived. It is very hard for night shift workers to get enough sleep during the day. They get a daily average of two to four hours less sleep than normal. Some researchers think it may take as long as three years to adjust to a shift work schedule. Others believe you will never fully adjust to an unusual sleep/wake pattern. Even if this is the case, you can make the best of a bad situation to sleep better.[35]

Cops work the overnight shift for a variety of reasons: low seniority, family advantages, less traffic, mostly hot calls, fewer report calls, and maybe no administrators around. But the overnight shift can have significant negative consequences for both the cop and his family. According to Howell and Nelson, "Health and wellbeing depends on social support and working overnights can be socially isolating, like you are living in a parallel universe."[36] Some cops coming off working the overnight shift can feel reborn, more human. One remarked to me, "I didn't realize that I was living constantly with a sort of low-grade headache."

Our circadian rhythm is our sleep/wake cycle, basically a 24-hour internal clock that cycles between sleepiness and wakefulness. This rhythm has been part of human biology for thousands of years, and it is best to work with it, not against it. The circadian system sets the window for the best sleep (the best sleep will be within that window of time), sleep outside the window will more likely be light, restless, with disturbing dreams, and waking.[37]

Everyone has a natural circadian rhythm that makes him or her either a morning or night person (or somewhere in between). According to sleep specialist Roxanne Prichard, to determine if you are a morning or evening person ask yourself "when is the best time for me to be awake and when is the best time for me to problem solve? If this is in the morning, you are a morning person and if in the afternoon and evening, you are a night person."[38]

Humans are essentially day creatures, some are early day people, some late day people, very, very few are so-called true night people. It is easier for a late day person to work the night shift. They can stretch their natural tendency. Night shift is very hard for morning people; however, if you are under forty it is much easier to tolerate the night shift. In a study of new police officers sleep response to shift work, the results suggested, "It may be possible to detect and even predict sleep deficiencies in response to shift work early on, which could be a basis for the development of individualized interventions to improve shift work tolerance."[39] Ideally, agencies would take this into consideration when assigning shift work.

Shift Work Sleep Disorder

Shift work sleep disorder, sometimes called shift work disorder or circadian rhythm sleep disorder, occurs when workers try to "sleep during a time that does not match with what their internal clock (circadian) is telling them to.

Shift Work Sleep Tips. Besides the basic tips mentioned earlier, here are some specific tips for those doing shift work:

- Take control of whatever part of your schedule you can, and try to adapt a strategy for optimal sleep.

- Strategic napping right before work, or during work for about 15 to 20 minutes to feel alert again. Or nap for up to 90 minutes if your home schedule permits.

- Use bright light treatment to manage your light-dark cycle by exposing yourself to bright light in the evening or first part of the night. Additionally, avoid bright light in the morning, which may include wearing sun glasses as you head home from work.

- A cool, quiet, dark sleep environment can be created using black-out curtains, ear plugs, white-noise machine, fans and temperature controls.

- Caffeine should be avoided prior to going to sleep and can be used strategically to aid in wakefulness.

- Exercise and eat well

Melatonin

There is no perfect sleep aid; however, some have found melatonin can be helpful, especially when transitioning between time zones or off-hour sleep that occurs when out of synch with circadian rhythm. Melatonin is a hormone that is produced normally at night and is suppressed by light exposure. Melatonin is available as an oral supplement.

All these tips might sound useless, especially when you are a new cop working odd hours with small children at home. But if you are a new cop working odd hours with small children at home, you have to know there are serious consequences of being less than alert or propped up with energy drinks. All things considered, making good sleep hygiene a priority and seeking treatment for chronic sleep problems is smart. Sleep is an important issue for everyone's wellness, but as police officers we have a culture of undervaluing it. There are many factors we cannot control with shift work, but the one thing we can do is to make sleep a priority and do all of the small accommodations in our life to make sure we get the best sleep we can.

It is common for cops and citizens alike to end interaction with the send-off, "Be safe." When cops say it, I think it is a reminder to be vigilant; for citizens, I think it is an expression of affection. Being safe or careful is good advice, but it cannot be our top priority because it requires taking more of a defensive posture. If you truly wished to be safe, better to stay behind hard cover all tour. I have advised young officers that when they hear "be safe," they can make the mental conversion to "be alert." Being alert allows for both safety and assertiveness. The primary contributor to our alertness is good sleep.

PART II

HARM AND HELP

TAKING CARE OF YOUR MENTAL HEALTH is as important as taking care of your physical health. However, the related *do's* and *don'ts* for physical health may seem more tangible. Mental health can feel harder to grasp. If mental health "illness" or "injury" were like a sore trigger finger, impacting our ability to do the job, or clumsily getting in the way while off-duty, it would be easier to deal with. But instead it is more often like a low-grade fever or malaise — a general feeling of discomfort, illness, or uneasiness whose exact cause is difficult to identify.[1]

Mental health troubles, from low mood to diagnosable depression, can be very unsettling, in part because we fear they have arrived to stay, this is our new life. Just that fear alone can make it worse. Likely these troubles are temporary, and in many cases, necessary. It may be helpful and more accurate to describe these things as *periods* of low-mood, or a *period* of depression, or a *period* of poor mental health. If that period lasts longer than you think is reasonable, or does not improve over time or with your best efforts, it still does not mean it is your new normal, but it could mean you need some kind of additional help. Try to not make it worse by isolating yourself from trusted others or taking unhealthy shortcuts to feeling different, by such means as drinking alcohol, having affairs, or excessively playing video games. The list of maladaptive coping is long, and if the urge is there, a healthy first step is to at least pause before you act and ask yourself, "What am I feeling?"

Officers must be alert to the early signs of mental and emotional trouble. There is a hazard of letting problems get really bad and then doing just enough to turn the pain volume down a notch while leaving the core issues unaddressed, instead of doing the necessary work to address the problem more thoroughly and completely. It can be very difficult for all people, and especially police officers, to acknowledge their vulnerabilities and reach out for help. A person can be great cop and contribute to a positive work atmosphere, but also have significant personal issues and struggles. We can help by decreasing the stigma of mental or emotional distress and providing education about recognizing trouble and getting appropriate help for it.

3 Columns of Officer Distress

Officers can experience a wide range of mental and emotional distress throughout their career. I have discovered, through my work as EAP Director, that this distress can often be sorted into one of three categories, with the understanding that sometimes there are interrelated or co-occurring problems. I created the *3 Columns of Officer Distress*™ to help me coordinate how best to respond, as well as actions to take to prevent some problems. Some of the distress or the events that cause the distress are unique to public safety work. Chapters 5, 6, and 7 will address each of these columns.

1. **Critical Incidents and Traumatic Events** are work-related events that temporarily overwhelm coping mechanisms.

2. **General Mental and Emotional Distress** are the range of psychological problems that all humans may suffer.

3. **Behavioral Health Crisis** is a loss of psychological function required to do the work.

I came up with these definitions on my own and you may notice they have a positive spin on them. For example, Critical Incidents and Traumatic Events, could have instead been defined as *"Bad things that happen to you at work that will scar you for life"*; General Mental and Emotional Distress, *"What's wrong with you"*; and Behavioral Health Crisis as, *"You can't be a cop anymore!"* I have found that if people are aimed toward the negative, especially if they are struggling or are in distress, that is where it seems they will go. Depression for example, can feel like a fog

3 Columns of Officer Distress

	Critical Incidents & Traumatic Events	General Mental & Emotional Distress	Behavioral Health Crisis
Definition	Work-related events that temporarily overwhelm coping mechanisms	The range of psychological problems that all humans may suffer	A loss of psychological function required to do the work
	Law Enforcement Specific	*Not Necessarily Law Enforcement Specific*	
Examples	Critical Incidents: • Officer-involved shooting • In-custody or enforcement action resulting in high probability of death, or death • Death or serious injury of coworker, Mass Casualty Event Traumatic Events: • "Bad calls"	• Anxiety and depression • Family and relationship conflicts • Sleep problems • Loss and grief • Work stress and frustration • Injury, illness and chronic pain • Substance misuse • Financial and legal concerns • Other and co-occurring conditions	May or may not include: • Severe depression • Mental health hospitalization • Suicide intention or attempt • Substance use disorder (detoxification or treatment facility admission)
	Post Traumatic Stress & Posttraumatic Stress Disorder		

in which your ability to see anything good is greatly diminished or absent. A hopeful message, encouragement and sometimes specific advice, can be most helpful. So how we define these things influences how we think about them.

I recognize this chart is anecdotal and simply a way to organize a police EAP response. Anytime you organize something as complex as human distress, there is a risk the organization may be subject to other interpretations. Furthermore, I included Post Traumatic Stress (PTS) and Posttraumatic Stress Disorder (PTSD) in this chart under all three columns because PTS/PTSD can easily fit into any and all three columns for a variety of reasons. Psychological trauma and PTS/PTSD will be discussed in Chapter 5.

CHAPTER 5

CRITICAL INCIDENTS AND TRAUMATIC EVENTS

Flash Bang

Definitions and Concepts

Critical incidents can be defined in a variety of ways. In law enforcement, a **critical incident** is a police action that is associated with or the cause of a death, significant or great bodily harm. This can also include intentional discharge of a firearm. These events are specific to our job and a known risk of police work.

A critical incident is most often obvious and on the extreme end of police work experience, such as shooting someone. These events impact both the officer and the agency, and rightly have many administrative implications or demands. With agency self-preservation in mind, police administrators define critical incidents primarily for the need of the agency, not necessarily the needs of the officers. One point of view could be that critical incidents are just traumatic events with more liability.

All other significant psychological traumas that do not meet the criteria of a critical incident might be categorized as **traumatic events**. However, traumatic events can be very difficult, maybe even impossible to define, in part because they can be so individualized, in which different events can have very different meanings for different people. Thus, I use the general description, "bad calls," for lack of a better term. Common themes that make for a "bad call" are things such as surprise, gore, or harm to an innocent person such as a child.

We certainly can think of examples, such as responding to a child struck and killed by a car, combined with the emotional intensity of a distraught driver or family members on scene. For most of us, that would be a psychologically traumatic event. Just discussing the topic of bad calls can lead any of us to bring to mind a particularly painful career event, an image or sound we likely will never forget. In all my years working in public safety, the most psychologically traumatic event for me was a death notification I did as an experienced officer, where I had to wake a child to tell him that his parents were dead. Like so many calls, it went relatively unnoticed by anyone else but the dispatcher who sent me.

We might be surprised by what we may have thought was a relatively small event or that a specific detail sticks with us. One cop described to me how a child looked at him and said, "I wish you were my dad." At the same time a cop could be in an officer-involved shooting and feel a cool detachment or a dispassionate reaction at the sight of someone they just killed lying on the ground. None of these reactions are necessarily right or wrong, good or bad. Some cops can feel bad for not feeling bad. It all depends, if something gets your attention, at some point you might want to explore it.

What once may have been referred to as a bad or shitty call may now be formally identified as a critical incident, traumatic event or other terms. This likely was an important effort to recognize it, to illuminate the idea that there can be harm associated with attending to the harm of others. However, the harm can be hard to predict and with a desire to detect and attend to harm, there is also a risk of over-reach or creating new expectations and unhealthy dependence. It may not be helpful or desirable to have an EAP, Critical Incident Stress Management (CISM) or therapeutic response for every, to put it crudely, dead baby call. Police work can be ugly; we need not act like bad things are not part of the job. Simultaneously we must recognize as psychologist George Bonanno has cautioned, "Events are not traumatic until we experience them as traumatic." They are potentially traumatic, but not automatically traumatic.[1]

I have a concern about the potential to over-diagnose PTSD[2] that stems from a desire to find a reason for our distress. Officers and their agencies must avoid being trendy and be careful not to first, find a label and second, cram people into it. For example, PTSD cannot be diagnosed immediately after a critical incident. One of the criteria of PTSD is the symptoms must last more than 1 month. On the other hand, post traumatic stress (PTS) following a critical incident could be a very reasonable, expected and a normal response. Being too eager to render a diagnosis or label something as abnormal is not helpful and can lead to other problems. I do not expect to leave this career without a few scratches and dents, and I believe I might have a touch of the old shellshock myself, but that is what can happen when you serve others and are up close to their suffering. And I do not want some of those memories or even the associated pain to go away. Good police work involves suffering. It is not necessarily about avoiding all suffering, but instead suffering better as needed.

With some caution about pathologizing trauma, we recognize that some critical incidents or traumatic events can be particularly mentally and emotionally troublesome for a variety of reasons. My brother, now a retired police officer, once told the story of having to use the fire department's pike pole to roll the severed head of a young woman out of a culvert. This was before I was a cop and I thought at the time, "Cops see and do extreme things, and sometime they go beyond the extreme." Examples of things that can "slip past our armor" and sneak or push past our defenses are those that surprise us, are particularly gruesome, involve innocence such as children, or for whatever reason are more personal. This can result in an immediate Acute Stress Reaction or Disorder, and if the condition were to go unresolved or get compounded by more psychological trauma, it could eventually result in PTSD.

I most certainly do not want to be accused of denying PTSD or minimizing people's suffering from psychological trauma. However, I do want to get our aim right, and not over-emphasize or misdirect our concern precisely because it can misdirect education and resources for those who do suffer persistent negative effects from psychological trauma. If you have experienced critical incidents or traumatic events yourself, or spoken to those who have, or been part of debriefings, you will note that it was not always the event that was so harmful but instead the feeling of being overwhelmed or helpless during the event that appears to be wounding. It is the rumination that does not allow you to leave it behind.

An agency cannot reliably detect when a critical incident or potentially traumatic event has had significant negative impact on an officer. What is more reliable and sustainable is helping officers recognize signs of distress in themselves or coworkers. Officers need to know that although they may suffer, they need not suffer alone. Agencies should reinforce long-standing organic systems of watching out for each other as well as mental health services that are accessible, efficient and trustworthy.

"That Was F'd Up"

Not all critical incidents or traumatic events are traumatic, and even if they are, we need not overreact. My observation about disturbing or upsetting-type calls, and I have heard others describe this as well, is that about two-thirds of public safety workers suffer little to no negative impact. They may feel bad for a while as they carry on, maybe preferring to stay busy with the next call for service or healthfully distract themselves from thoughts of it while the experience fades into the past. The reason I emphasize *healthfully* is because responding by stuffing it down, drinking to avoid uncomfortable thoughts and emotions, or any number of actions or inaction may help in the short term, but these actions may have their own negative consequences including preventing healthy processing.

About one-third of officers will be negatively impacted. A percentage of those will be fine with time, and the other percent will feel stuck and may need extra time or some help working through it. The difference between the "bad call" they never forget, and those they do, may be a matter of degrees, or could be thought of as a continuum from bad to worse. Identifying which events will be problematic can be both an art and science, and any attempt to strictly define them based on the incident or as an outsider looking in, is likely impossible. A cop can be right in the middle of a critical incident and have little to no negative psychological impact, while the most impacted officer will be someone on the periphery. Maybe the event has more personal meaning for them, or they were the dispatcher, or an officer who had to listen to a cop pleading for help over the radio and could not get to the scene. A clinician may at some later point be able to identify the level of impact, but it can be hard for others and maybe even the impacted cop to know. An immediate clue that a particular event or call was impactful might be heard in cop language, "Well, that was fucked up."; or "What just happened?"; or expressing a strong reaction or anger on scene, but who is to say these officers are not better off for doing more immediate processing. In fact, feeling bad about bad things is not bad. When your fellow officers acknowledge something was a big deal, signaling that it was impactful, it can make the event feel less like a personal big deal by making it a shared experience.

There is a new factor in police work, body worn cameras (BWCs), and the impact on officer-to-officer interactions is not yet known. Body worn cameras interfere with the mini-debriefs that officers do naturally after each call, the seemingly casual conversation that occurs when things have wrapped up. I would call this an unintended consequence. While the cops could coordinate amongst themselves an 'all-clear" to talk signal, it is easier to just walk away or drive off without the huge benefit of talking with each other. I believe the biggest harm from BWCs is how unnatural it makes our ability to communicate, the one thing that makes humans unique and more successful than any other creature on earth. There are benefits to BWCs to be sure, but unintended consequences as well. Cops will adapt as they do; I encourage them as well as agency leaders to make post-event communication a priority.

Potentially Traumatic Events

Our best chance of helping officers who suffer the flash bang or slow burn of psychological trauma is to have a category of potentially traumatic events. With this, we do our best to identify them and it gives us a systematic way to attend to all the "bad calls." The difficulty comes in identifying them. This is where pre-event education, peer support, and informed supervision can be very helpful, as well as emphasizing officers' personal responsibility to seek help if time does not heal as expected. Even if we miss some events, the existence of the "bad calls" category alerts cops to the potential harm of such events.

When I was new in my EAP job, my boss asked me to write a traumatic event policy. I thought about it and came back to our next meeting and said, "How about we don't.", not in a flip way, but in a strategic way. A policy poorly written, or written for the wrong reason, can do more harm than good, including limiting options. Unlike critical incidents, most potentially traumatic events do not require specific administrative actions and can often be handled on a case-by-case basis. If you can identify officers impacted by an event, it may not matter if it was defined as a critical incident or traumatic event. At my agency, I have the ability to offer most, or all of the same, supportive and therapeutic services to those involved in a potentially traumatic event as to those involved in a critical incident.

No Head Shrinking, Thank You

The therapeutic services offered following a critical incident or traumatic event are supportive and psychoeducational to aid in the normalization and management of any acute stress response. These services are not intended to evaluate for Fitness for Duty. If the clinician discovers any serious concerns about the client's mental health or their ability to fully function in their assigned duty, it is their professional responsibility to act accordingly.

There should be no assumption that because an officer takes a police action he has trained for, maybe even rehearsed mentally, that he should be evaluated for his mental fitness. Routine fitness for duty evaluations of officers involved in shootings is contrary to both the Fitness for Duty and Officer Involved Shooting Guidelines made known by The International Association of Chiefs of Police.

Cops are suspicious creatures who primarily want to know that they are okay; these post-critical incident services will not function if officers believe that being honest about their distress could cost them their job. If we get this wrong, send mixed messages about mental health resources, it will fail or go unused. Doing the work that society asks of an officer, in particular being involved in deadly use of force, should not result in an officer having to prove his sanity.

Psychological Trauma

The things that harm or injure our body most likely cause pain, taste bad, or make us sick to our stomach. The events that harm or injure our mind may cause anxiety, depression or fear. The brain, as therapist Yoland Harper points out, "has a remarkable ability to link a current situation with anything that looks like, sounds like, smells like, taste like, or feels like a previous threatening situation. The brain feels unsafe so it reminds you of that prior event."[3]

Sebastian Yunger is a journalist, author and filmmaker who has embedded himself with combat soldiers and writes about PTSD in a way that makes me hang on his every word. Yunger has said that humans have evolved to deal with trauma. We are the descendants of people who acted well in a crisis or else we would not be here today[4]. In a 2015 article titled, *How PTSD Became a Problem Far Beyond the Battlefield,* he described his surprise experience with a panic attack and reaction to a psychological trauma this way, "From an evolutionary perspective, it's exactly the response you want to have when your life is in danger: you want to be vigilant, you want to react to strange noises, you want to sleep lightly and wake easily, you want to have flashbacks that remind you of the danger, and you want to be, by turns, anxious and depressed. Anxiety keeps you ready to fight, and depression keeps you from being too active and putting yourself at greater risk. This is a universal human adaptation to danger that is common to other mammals as well. It may be unpleasant, but it's preferable to getting eaten."[5]

Bessel van der Kolk, an authority on psychological trauma describes it as "an event that overwhelms the central nervous system and changes the way you remember and react to things that remind you of it." There are very bad events that you are incapable of assimilating and integrating into your life. They can include violent attacks or "being unseen and unprotected from harm or the experience of having to manage difficulty alone."[6]

Psychological trauma or stress can reveal itself in specific ways which the DSM-5 lists as the core PTSD symptoms:

> **Hyperarousal:** increases in heart rate, respiration and blood pressure; psycho-motor agitation, physical tension, difficulty sleeping, anxiety, fear, irritability or anger.

> **Avoidance:** avoiding exposure to the trauma, including talking about it, thinking about it, visiting the place where it occurred or seeing people who shared the experience of it; other avoidant symptoms might include withdrawing from friends and family, being unable to go back to work if it was an on-the-job trauma.

> **Intrusions:** intrusive thoughts or memories of the traumatic event; flashbacks, in which people feel as though they are reliving the event with great intensity, and nightmares.

> **Psychic numbing:** a sense of being emotionally numb after a trauma, experiencing a sense of unreality, dissociative amnesia, in which the traumatic event is pushed out of awareness, "spacing out" and using substances to "numb out."[7]

Human survival is dependent on the ability to link certain experiences, especially those that threaten us, with an emotion and store it as a memory. When faced with that experience again, it is useful to instantly recall the feeling. Cops are often quick-studies of human nature because our lives depend on the ability to recognize and respond to danger. Experienced cops can recognize a "gun face," the body language and facial expression given the officer by someone spotted illegally carrying a gun. Or the subtle differences in hand and arm movement when a suspect has something weighted, like a pistol, in their hand. Maybe below consciousness, at the gut level, the cop's response is a feeling somewhere between fear and thrill. What may be unhelpful, is feeling anxious, depressed, or fearful when there is no threat. And unless properly processed, psychologically traumatic experiences can get stuck, so to speak, and interfere with daily living.

The symptoms of psychological trauma occurring in childhood may differ from those occurring in adulthood, and those occurring as police officers may differ in some ways from those occurring as a soldier, EMT, paramedic, firefighter or other adults. It is possible that a police officer could suffer a single psychological trauma exposure related to an on-duty event, but it may be difficult to differentiate or separate that event from other life events or work incidents.

This has special relevance for police officers because of the mental and emotional harm that can come from the things we see and do, routine and not so routine. Cops can be well practiced in managing potent psychologically traumatic events because of their repeated exposure, an inoculation of sorts. But it is a matter of fact that psychological trauma can be extremely impactful, affecting us negatively in the moment, or seemingly by sneak attack after we thought we successfully stuffed it down and out of sight.

Fortunately, there are treatments and healing processes that are transformative and can help to disentangle painful emotions from the memory they are associated with. This is demonstrated when someone is able to talk about a really horrific thing, reflect on it, but not re-experience it. They still have the memory, but not the overwhelming emotion attached to it. Ideally, we want our past in our past, accessible as needed to inform us, but not to hostilely appear in our face, interfering with our present.

Big "T" and Little "t" Trauma

Just as with physical injury, not all psychological trauma is the same. Many in the psychological trauma field use the labels big "T" versus little "t" trauma to differentiate between the reaction to a single bad event and the reaction caused by multiple smaller events. For police officers, trauma is more incident-specific, big "T" trauma, as when an officer experiences someone else's death up close. Little "t" trauma could be the steady diet of victim and victimizer, repeatedly witnessing poverty, neglect and the suffering of others. In police work, little "t" trauma is much more common, but less dramatic, and possibly over time more harmful. For the so-called normal, healthy, and relatively safe citizen, big "T" could be a car crash, little "t" could be a citation from a grumpy cop.

Among police officers, we tend to focus on big "T" trauma, and probably will continue to, but it is the little "t" trauma that is much more common. The big "T" traumas stand out and really get your attention; the repeated little "t" traumas can leave us feeling helpless and hopeless. I recall a moment like this, I was gathering information and making plans to have a dull-eyed child placed into protective custody when the sloppy drunk and high mother blurted out that she was pregnant. I just hung my head in resignation.

Some traumas slip past your armor or pierce the armor and rattle around inside the hard shell, by being so horrific or by surprising you. Understanding how the brain works when it perceives danger can help you understand why a critical incident can feel like a mysterious force that has taken you on a wild ride.

How the Brain Works

Our Animal Brain and Human Brain

The brain can be grouped into three parts:

1. Reptilian (brain stem)

2. Mammalian (midbrain)

3. Human (forebrain)

For greater simplicity, we can group the reptilian and mammalian brain and call it the **animal brain**, because like animals, it is more basic or instinctual and about the size of your thumbs. The **human brain** is probably what we think of when we visualize the brain (the *you* that makes you *you*). Our human brain is huge, about the size of your two fists, which when pressed together, resembles the two lobes of the brain. The human brain can be further described as the conscious brain, thinking brain, big brain, or outer brain. The animal brain is located at the top of your spinal cord, at the base of your forebrain. Other descriptors for the animal brain could be the subconscious brain, reactive brain, little brain, lower brain, or inner brain. Evolutionarily, the animal brain is older, more basic, whereas the human, or forebrain, is newer and fancier and appears as if it grew out of the midbrain, which grew out of the brain stem.

Animal Brain (Brain Stem & Midbrain)	Human Brain (Forebrain)
Subconscious brain	Conscious brain
Reacting brain	Thinking brain
Little brain	Big brain
Inner brain	Outer brain
Older, more basic brain	Newer and fancier brain
Reptilian or mammalian brain	Modern or human brain

A reasonable response to extreme danger may be fight, flight, freeze, or even faint. All but fainting can be a conscious choice, but when seconds or fractions of seconds count, we can rely on our animal brain, and specifically the limbic area to save us. The limbic area turns thought down and action up. Within the limbic area is the amygdala, "a cluster of neurons in an almond shape that link a range of functions together, including responding directly to perceptual input, filtering incoming data for danger, scanning faces, remembering emotionally arousing events, and embedding traumatic events into memory to avoid trauma in the future. An overactive amygdala can be thought of as 'too differentiated' and create anxiety in our lives, that feeling of unspecified concern or dread that may have no thoughts, just a feeling. Trauma can increase amygdala firing and growth."[8]

The human brain is big and complex, a slow data processor compared to our animal brain. It is also flexible, meaning, it is able to interpret data allowing you to think differently about something, change your mind or get a new thought. The animal brain is ridged or inflexible. It processes signals at incredible speeds, without bias or interpretation to slow it down. The animal brain is designed for short-term survival and when we receive a danger signal for example, the human brain defers to the animal brain and will go "off-line" or power down so as not to interfere. The animal brain is always on, always working. It keeps us breathing, regulates temperature and is always on patrol for sudden immediate danger.

Which brain is in charge? It depends, of course, on whether you are reading a book or your child is in danger. Once, one of my children suffered a serious looking head laceration in a fall. I was not there, but my wife was. She told how she picked him up and began running. Later I asked her where she was running to, and she said, "I don't know." If a wild animal had caused the injury, she was fully prepared to claw it to death in defense with her bare hands or try to out run it. Reading these words, you are in your human brain, but if while reading there was a sudden loud crash, you might suddenly shift to your animal brain.

Let us revisit the garden hose-snake story in Chapter 2. Imagine you are working around your home and go into a garage or shed to retrieve a tool. In the dim light, you are suddenly faced with a coiled snake, reared up and ready to strike; maybe you even visualize being bitten. Literally, without thinking, you leap backwards to safety. In the bright light, and as you, "repopulate" your thinking brain, it slowly occurs to you that the snake was awfully green and located where you store your garden hose. Because your animal brain (fast, rigid, always on) cannot determine if your experience is real or imagined, and your human brain (slow and subservient) had shut down, you had the physical experience as if it were a real snake, even if it was a garden hose. But had it been a snake, thinking too much could have been a problem by slowing your response.

The unconscious mind arrives first, and the conscious mind is more of an observer of the feelings and sensations brought on by the unconscious. Your unconscious mind may make a decision that you give the conscious mind credit for.

Whether it is the human brain-animal brain fliparoo or the effects of some related chemical response, very dangerous, surprising, extreme or novel events can leave us feeling like our brain is playing tricks on us, and we are just passengers on a wild ride. Yet with experience or practice, as we might see with expert cops, athletes, sportsmen or skilled workers, some individuals flirt with harnessing these powers. When they do, we can see it in their faces as it takes on the appearance of being supremely focused, in the zone. Maybe this is what we see when cops put on their "game face", the relaxed, slightly absent look of seriousness when it is "go time." We might also see, in our coworkers (or the general public who are unaccustomed or unpracticed in routine danger) the wild or absent look in their eyes, babbling, or non-purposeful movement, as someone who is not in their human or thinking brain. This is easy to imagine if we envision the thinking brain as diminished or disconnected in relation to the animal brain during scary events. When I meet with cops after critical incidents, I am aware that sometimes they have not fully returned to their human brain or are still feeling the physical or chemical effects of the wild-ride.

It is helpful to know how the brain works during extreme events. I, like many, learned how the brain works the hard way, from direct experience and observation. Throughout my careers as an EMT, paramedic, and police officer, and my study of the topic, as well as someone who now meets with officers involved in such things as an officer-involved shooting within minutes to hours after the event, I have gained some insight into how the brain works.

Super Focus

Intense events, especially dangerous ones at work, require super focus. Super focus, or selective attention, by definition means you do not see or experience other nonessential things. A Lexipole report states, "There will be an immediate tendency to focus on the perceived threat, to the exclusion of all other stimuli. As a result, the officer may fail to perceive peripheral activities."[9] Officers and others can have unrealistic expectations about memory when involved in extreme events such as a shooting.

It is reasonable to expect they will be able to recall their primary focus but not peripheral information.

The tunnel vision, audio exclusion and time distortion can be scientifically explained and are related to this super focus and the human brain deferring to the animal brain. Interestingly, intense focus, such as while engaged in a hobby or personal interest such as fishing, hunting, gardening or woodworking can be very relaxing. Whereas super focus while at work when faced with danger, would not be considered relaxing.

Gaps and Crooked Lines

When the emergency part is all over, and you repopulate your full brain, "re-enter" or "return" to the human brain, there may be gaps and crooked lines in your memory. The altered sensations or sensory distortion can be unnerving and having just experienced possibly the biggest call of your career and not remembering how many bullets you fired or who was standing next to you can be upsetting. These voids do not remain empty or as the economist Geoffrey Crowther pointed out, "...the trouble about a vacuum is that it gets filled. And if there are no angels available to fill it, fools or worse rush in."[10] In other words, unless we recognize this, any self-doubt, distress or perceived criticism might lead us down a path of unfounded self-loathing.

When I explain that memory gaps or altered sensations can be a sign of a high-functioning brain, not a defective one, it can bring officers great relief. Additionally, the mind seems to need a sleep cycle or two to fully "recover,"[11] and some events will never be recalled. All this, especially the memory gaps, can be unnerving and problematic.

A strange and sometimes embarrassing experience during extreme events can be a dissociative moment. This is the experience of mentally leaving, where you might feel unhinged, untethered, your world spinning out of control, not necessarily in a dizzy sort of way, but as if you are losing contact with the world, as if your subconscious mind was saying, "I have to protect you. I'm getting you out of here." For example, cops sometimes see this disassociation when talking with victims of sexual violence, such as a child victim who because they could not physically escape the horror, did so mentally.

These events become memorable because, in addition to their intensity or novelty, it can be embarrassing to have tunnel vision, surprising to have a dissociative moment, frightening or mysterious to have gaps in your memory. I find it hard to believe that most cops, early in their career as they are training their brain, do not ask themselves at one point, "Am I defective? Maybe I'm not cut out for this work?" when they compare their novice insides to a veteran's outsides.

A more detailed explanation of the brain science behind these odd experiences may not be necessary, what is most helpful is just knowing there is an explanation for it and it is a normal reaction to an abnormal event. In other words, it has happened to other cops and you are okay.

Physical Response to Hyperarousal

When an immediate threat to our safety occurs, we become hyper-aroused, which instantly prepares us for a fight or flight. This is not something we think about, that would be too slow. Instead, there is a general discharge of the sympathetic nervous system. The resulting physical effects include physical changes and stress-induced distortions such as: heart and breathing rate increase, bladder relaxation, tunnel vision, shaking hands, dilated pupils, dry mouth, and hearing loss.

These physical effects, which can feel very strange, can all be explained physiologically, for example, tunnel vision or muffled or absent hearing is a result of selective attention, the tendency to focus on the perceived threat, to the exclusion of all other stimuli. Loss of motor skills can be related to a de-emphasis on fine motor movement in favor of gross motor movement like running or fighting.

My brother once told me a story of running his mouth in a bar and being called out into the alley to fight, he pissed his pants. I once saw a gang member with defensive stab wounds all over his hands and arms, he had shit his pants. As cops, we are highly motivated to avoid these responses — training, experience and a little Situational Self-Awareness can help.

Preparation For Traumatic Events: Situational Self-Awareness

I believe that with some self-awareness and practice, the harm, need-less discomfort, and confusion from critical incidents, traumatic events or otherwise extreme events could be lessened, and we could improve the speed and quality of normalization and recovery. Instead of solely attending to the distress following an event, we can take what some of us learned the hard way, and help others before, during and after. I call this **situational self-awareness.** It involves self-control in the form of managing our interpretation of events.

Before a Critical Incident: Pre-event Education

Be A Student of Yourself. New experiences can be very enlivening. Maybe the first time you drove a police car with red lights and siren it was thrilling, but gradually it became routine. By definition, novel things are new, and it may not be fully possible to prepare for extreme novelty. But with experience, practice and study, novel events in effect gradually decrease, yet do not disappear, as can be recognized in the statement, "Well, I thought I'd seen it all." Effective police work is a craft where one experience builds on the next. Undoubtedly, the first time you went "hands-on" with a bad guy, you learned tons from the real-life application of control tactics, what worked, what did not. Maybe you defaulted to fighting as if you were drunk in a bar, but that was a lesson too. As a carpenter learns the nature of his tools and wood, we learn the nature of both the criminal and ourselves. No two police calls are ever identical, but the one constant is that *you* are there. People who fail to learn from experience often lack self-awareness; we can be a student of ourselves. Learning how your brain works, and how your body responds to extreme intensity and stress helps you know what to expect in yourself and others.

Because you cannot always have direct experience, nor do you want to, you practice. In lieu of, or in addition to practice, you can employ mental rehearsal in the forms of imaging and visualization. You can train the brain to be accustomed to the possibilities of extreme events, both vicariously through observation and shared stories or mental rehearsal.

Be Alert. Advantage yourself by operating from a position of strength by being alert, physically fit, well-rested, and well-fed. Good health and wellbeing will help you not only perform better, and recover quicker, but also makes you less vulnerable to the negative effects of these experiences. Being alert can minimize the element of surprise; a common theme of those negatively impacted by psychological trauma is that it caught them off guard.

Conserve Your Energy. Day to day you can conserve your mental and emotional energy by acting purposefully to protect yourself and minimize exposure to certain images, conversations, or people that are unhappy and want to share that unhappiness. Off-duty this can include avoiding or seeking balance with social media. On-duty, most cops reach a point where they limit the images they add to their mental library. If you do not have to view a dead body, and you do not want to see the dead body, avoid the dead body. Conserving emotional energy can include avoiding vigorous complaining, you know very well that bitching and complaining can feel very satisfying, enjoyable, and in some cases build rapport, but it takes a lot of emotional energy, most often leaving you feeling worse for it.

During and Immediately After a Critical Incident

If during big "T" trauma or a critical incident your animal brain (subconscious) is in charge, and your human brain (conscious) has gone off-line, how will you know that you are in an extreme event? What is your mental awareness, and how does it feel? Some people experience a single-minded focus. Others may experience a sensation of falling down a hole, or the world starting to spin, or the thought that they are losing their mind or grip on reality. More likely, you will feel that you are somewhere in-between the two brains.

Battle of the Brains. Once as a young EMT, I was trapped in a house, hiding in a bathroom from a knife-wielding madman. Searching for an escape route I passed a mirror and saw my own face, it looked terrified. Climbing out a second-floor window, I recall repeating to myself, *"This is real. This is really happening!"* I felt actively involved in a battle between the two brains.

The animal brain has our best interests in mind, but eventually people need to get back home to their thinking brain, to get the whole brain working again. We sometimes clumsily navigate new experiences, sometimes masterfully, artfully using our body language, and our words so as to decrease real or imagined danger and fear. De-escalation is not a new concept for cops. It is something we do every day in patrol work, helping people reengage the rational brain. We apply it in the toughest situations on the street. Just as we might give a hysterical person a few simple specific instructions, such as telling them they are safe now and to breath, we can do the same to coworkers or ourselves. You can interrupt your own doomsday thinking and deliberately calm yourself, even in the midst of a crisis.

Giving yourself a pep talk helps, but what if you are not in the mood or state of mind to listen? The stressed mind needs simple direction, not a lot of talk, so the things that help are simple as well, like a big arrow pointing you in the direction of the thinking brain. At a gut level, certain activities, habits and routines, signal the human brain that you are ready to return partially or fully. These are things that indicate to the brain relative safety or can at least be employed to cajole your brain into thinking so, such as controlled breathing, purposeful talking, seeing a calm face, and drinking water.

Breathing. The freeze part of fight, flight, freeze, faint, might include holding your breath, but holding one's breath and the related lack of oxygen will likely make things worse. The act of breathing, especially slow deep full breaths seems to be a special link or bridge between the mind and body. Controlled breathing cannot only break the trance, but as SWAT and snipers know, is a useful tool for managing mind and body.

Talking. You have certainly heard talking that sounds a lot like babbling, or compressed speech that is high pitched as a result of extreme duress. In these cases, the person may not even know what they are saying. But controlled purposeful commands, instruction or helpful self-talk can engage your breathing and brain. Even joking can be useful. Many of us can recall being in a tense situation when some cop said something hilariously inappropriate, but helpful. This may have caused us to realize that they had mastery over their own brain, cutting the tension by breathing and activating the thinking brain.

Unless they prefer it, do not expect a cop to sit down or stand still immediately following an intense event. Some have recognized the value in what has been called the hot walk and talk, where moving while talking (or not talking) helps settle them down.

Self-Talk. Employing such phrases as "I can handle this" or banishing the opposite, "I can't handle this," can act as internal encouragement. And consider what was covered in Chapter 2 about the stress narrative and making stress your friend.

Calm Face. A calm or friendly face, maybe someone you know calling your name can signal safety. I did something similar to this routinely as a paramedic, knowing that sick and injured people often judged the severity of their condition by my reaction to it.

Drinking Water. Without thinking, drinking water sends signals from the gut to the brain that you are safe, or relatively so. Probably because your ancient self knows that if you were in mortal danger, you would not be drinking or eating stuff. Your gut does the thinking and signals the all-clear for you. My first sergeant told me that he used to have a bottle of water in his squad for just that purpose, his instincts told him this would help a cop feel normal again.

Noticing Physical Sensations. When feeling stressed, whether you are qualifying at the gun range, or in the midst of a critical incident, it is useful to recognize the physical sensations are there on your behalf, and see them as your friend, not your enemy. Rather than totally trying to rid yourself of them, you can see them as making you more alert and part of peak performance.

Immediately after a traumatic event, being near supportive others may be all we need, and humans have probably intuitively understood this throughout history. Additionally, as our understanding of psychological trauma continues to evolve, we will discover other helpful practices and procedures to mitigate the harm when the brain is most vulnerable or raw if you will, and the debris is still settling. Blocking certain types of memory formation may be a way to prevent PTSD in some situations. The memory consolidation process can take hours to days to complete, and it may be possible to either prevent or weaken traumatic memories during a window of time immediately following a psychologically traumatic event.[12] This could involve certain medications or other deliberate practices.

In the mid-2000s, I was involved in an officer-involved shooting. While segregated with my monitoring officer awaiting the completion of the administrative process, I recalled an article I had read some time earlier about experimenting with distracting the recently traumatized brain by having people play the video game Tetris.[13] I found a computer but was unable to load a game of Tetris, so instead I played several hands of guilt-free solitaire on work time. I do not know what effect it had other than projecting an image of cold-blooded killer. Recently, I have initiated at my agency another idea, bringing in comfort dogs for cops to interact with while processing traumatic events. I have also purchased a hand-held Tetris game for our department.

After a Critical Incident

Immediately after a critical incident, the same things apply, controlled breathing, purposeful talking, seeing a calm face, and drinking water, help the officer transition back into his thinking brain, if he is not there already. In theory, water can be additionally helpful by flushing out stress toxins. Some may go home, sleep fine, and be fully recovered and ready to return to work the next day. For others, even if uncomplicated by other factors, it could take the body and mind days and a few sleep cycles to fully recover. If complicated by physical injury, legal or policy concerns, administrative conflict, or psychological trauma, full recovery could take much longer.

Following a critical incident, it is not uncommon for an officer to recollect a recent or particularly troublesome past event, like adding up the hard miles on a car. It is not clear to me if psychological trauma or even stress accumulates — maybe instead it is a lack of full recovery from previous events. Too much trauma in close proximity can feel like accumulation. Though I am concerned for officers, I do not find it helpful to make any assumptions that they have been harmed by their psychological trauma exposure or that they have not successfully faced more difficult events in their careers or personal lives. If they may be harmed, the purpose of after-care is to assure that they normalize as quickly and efficiently as possible. What may have surprised them often does not surprise me. I remind them that with time, officers almost always get better on their own; however, sometimes they take an unnecessarily long route to get there, unprocessed trauma can make you feel stuck. We learn to be cops through experience. Critical incidents are most often unique and surprising events, and the officers themselves may not know what they need to fully recover. Sometimes our best effort is aimed at supporting them as they figure it out.

Short Term. In police work we look for trouble and sometimes find it, or it finds us. The job can be boring and then suddenly intense or life threatening. Many armed encounters, for example, can go from investigating someone or something suspicious to self-defense within seconds. Following an intense event, the involved officer can suddenly feel like they are being treated as if they are compromised. Administrative processes take them from warrior to "wounded," and they are now being cared for. This can be a very unwanted, unnatural feeling and run contrary to how they expect to be treated. Despite what an officer may want, and especially in the chaotic aftermath of some of these scenes, it is likely in everyone's best interest to order an officer to comply with critical incident protocols and routines. But understand that if the crisis is still ongoing or they feel like it is, it may be difficult and insulting to make them stand-down, sometimes a good compromise is to reassign them to something behind enemy lines so to speak.

Recovery starts when we get out of the kill-zone and start to transition out of the police role. It may take returning home and interacting with loved ones before an officer can more fully appreciate that they have been impacted by the incident. Interestingly, I once spoke with an officer who lived alone. He told me that following his shooting, he asked a buddy to tactically search his house before he went in.

In the short-term, partial recovery might be the best you should expect. During troubled times, you might settle for some amount of good rest and revitalization. It reminds me of when our kids were small, especially when some or all of us were sick. My wife and I would go to bed thinking, "If we could just get a few hours of sleep, we'll be okay. We can make it." In police terms, it might mean, just recovering some of your strength. You might seek a literal nap or a figurative nap; most important is to make healthy choices. Zoning-out in front of a sports channel while ignoring your family may not be ideal, but it is better than drinking. Ideal would be some good sleep, exercise, a good laugh with your family and friends. If you are struggling with intrusive images, anger, or sleep problems to name a few, get help processing it through peer support, therapeutic help or trusted friends. One cop told me that after particularly bad calls, she holds it together until her drive home, and after really bad ones, she gives herself a day to get over it. She had called me when she had not gotten "over it" as she was accustomed. To me that is resiliency and smart self-care. As stated earlier regarding the benefit of helpful self-talk during the event, after the event you can also tell yourself such things as "I did a good job" or "I'll know better next time."

Long Term. Following big "T" trauma, it can be hard to know *why* you are negatively impacted. For some, you might be surprised by how you feel or thought you would feel back to normal by now. Some might be easily startled, angry and defensive with the loved ones, have sleep troubles or even flashbacks. Symptoms that continue after weeks or months may need some specialized therapeutic attention.

There can be long-term or lingering effects of psychological trauma or more precisely, a lack of full recovery. There are many among us who have suffered psychological trauma as a child or adult and continue to have profound problems. Try as they might, suppressing does not seem to fully work, though the attempt is respectable. In the film *Band of Brothers*, the production included interviews with actual WWII veterans. These men, who returned home, raised children, worked entire careers and constantly contributed to their community, can be seen suddenly crying as they touch on thoughts and images from their war past. The memory is still linked with the original emotion. Whether a veteran, cop, adults with adverse childhood experiences, having past events increasingly come into your consciousness, does not need to be viewed as bad, likely it is a sign of life progress, not regress. Possibly now, more than ever before, you are finally ready to give it the attention it needs, professionally or otherwise.

Supervisor's Role In Critical Incidents

On-Scene Supervisor Role

Immediately following a critical incident, such as an officer-involved shooting, scene supervision is critical, and aside from assigning someone to stay with the involved officer (monitoring officer), agencies do well to stay focused on police procedures and not involve EAP or necessarily seek EAP-like resources at this time. I believe that during the first half-hour or more of a critical incident it is preferable for cops to stay in their cop brain, not thinking or feeling too much, and certainly not talking freely about the event.

Beyond, "Are You Okay?" .

Approaching an officer after a critical incident or a bad call and asking "Are you okay?" is generally understood as a signal that the supervisor recognizes the potential for a negative mental and emotional impact from the event. However, do not expect an honest answer. An officer may not want to, need to, or be ready to process an event. And a response of, "I'm good," may mean they are fine or they expect to be. But it may also be too soon to tell, and this is not the time or place to try to figure that out. Asking is a reasonable gesture, and an important indication that the supervisor cares, but supervisors may need to go beyond just asking.

An understanding of how the brain works and what disassociation can look like is an important supervisory skill. Extreme events can create a battle of the brains, leaving an officer somewhere between the midbrain and forebrain as well as have residual physical effects related to adrenaline. Disassociation is the experience of mentally leaving the current reality and is most often detected in others by an absent look in the eyes, lack of focus, or difficulty with speech. The best help a supervisor can give is to signal the "all-clear" by remaining calm and confident herself and "talking" directly to the brain stem and midbrain via the gut by having the officer drink water and take slow full breaths if warranted.

Strong reactions on scene can be a good thing from a speed of recovery point-of-view, but open expressions of grief or anger can alarm other officers. It is not uncommon for witness officers or supervisors to ask me to check on an officer who had a strong reaction, only for me to find they appear to be have managed it well, that the emotion "had its say" and moved on, like something that passed through them as opposed to getting stuck.

We may recognize that someone is disassociating or not functioning well. In those cases it may be better to assign someone to share their responsibility or gently relieve them of their duties by giving them a lesser task, rather than asking too much about how they feel. A respectful approach can be to ask them, "What do you think you need right now?"

If an officer were to decompensate for whatever reason, start to have some kind of mental or emotional response, the on-scene supervisor, fellow officers, and peer support can step in to console him as needed. Even if specialized supportive or therapeutic people were requested to the scene, they could not be relied upon to arrive on scene in a timely manner and expecting their help may undermine an expectation that supervisors and fellow officers are responsible to each other for mental and emotional support. Additionally, a critical incident scene is about street cops doing what street cops do best and supervisors supervising. EAP-like intervention may not be wanted, needed or appropriate just yet.

A cop once told me that after his shooting, the others cops gathered around him, first checked him for holes, then hustled him off to a squad where they sat him in the passenger seat, cranked up the air-conditioning and handed him a bottle of water. In this case, the officer felt indebted to the other cops and their instincts to protect him that way. Another cop described getting a big *I'm-glad-you-are-not-dead* hug from a big bear of a cop.

There is no perfect response to cover all situations, but we should at least know what not to do, that is allow a cop to remain isolated. Most cops can recall a scene or a story of a shooter-officer left sitting alone on a curb or what have you, because people were so freaked out and unsure of what to do. Mammals need to be near others when wounded.

Monitoring Officer

At my agency, involved officers are paired with what we call a *monitoring officer*. Other agencies that have formalized this role may have other names for this. The on-scene supervisor, or even a senior officer, will assign each involved officer his own monitoring officer. The purpose and function are both protective and humane. They remain together at all times, except when the involved officer is meeting with his attorney or investigator. The monitoring officer and the involved officer do not talk about the incident. This practice is very useful, and like many things, it was born out of need, a need to humanely and legally protect officers and the agency. It is not complex, and some officers perform this role naturally, but officers and supervisors need training in what this role is and is not.

It can be very unnatural to limit contact with, and free expression between, officers following what may have been the most intense experience of their career. An involved officer and his partner may have gone to academy together, spend 8 or 10 hours a day responding to calls together or in some cases share a squad car. They may spend more time with each other than they do their spouses, then suddenly they are in a shootout, and moments later not allowed to talk with each other or other friends and coworkers; this feels very unnatural.

No assumption should be made that the involved officer has done anything wrong, or if he may have done something wrong, no assumption that it was ill intended. It also should not be assumed that the officer is mentally or physically compromised by the event, but he could be, so the monitoring officer acts as a protector from any physical or legal harm. Furthermore, the involved officer becomes a critical piece of evidence, who must have their integrity and chain of custody, so to speak, protected, as they may be asked to account for all of their post-event actions and interactions. Additionally, the monitoring officer acts as a barrier, cautioning the officer not to talk about the event and keeping others away so they do not talk about the event to them. So, the best way to protect the officer is to separate them out and strictly limit their access to others. A monitoring officer's purpose is not intended to be therapeutic, but a buddy of sort, to help them be quiet and calm. We assign another cop to stand with them because it is important they are not isolated or given the impression that separating them is because they did something wrong.

When the involved officer and his monitoring officer are released from the scene, together they go directly to a designated waiting area, headquarters for example. There they wait together through the rest of the process. The monitoring officer role can be applied in other situations as well, anytime an officer is in severe distress for whatever reason.

Allowing for Recovery to Start

If a supervisor is concerned about the impact of any call on an officer or group of officers, the supervisor has a number of options that range from ignoring it, to treating it like a critical incident and seeking CISM (Critical Incident Stress Management) resources.

The supervisor can also simply visit with the officers and talk about it. Having a supervisor or senior officer acknowledge the potential harm from the ugly sights and sounds of police work can send an important message that it is okay to feel the impact of a sad or bad event. This could include a small-group meeting or private one-on-one check-ins.

The supervisor may need to nudge the cops away from a critique of tactics or politics, and guide them towards a conversation about any strong reactions or concerns. Following some situations, such as when a child was killed or injured, officers may need some time expressing anger and frustration. A question that can get a conversation going can be, "What was the worst part about this event for you?" At the very least, the intent is to acknowledge the mental and emotional distress. The supervisor can say she is concerned about the officer's wellbeing and wants to provide help with recovery.

Recovery might be a brief talk here and now or a follow-up session with a peer support team member. It could include a referral to an EAP resource if the officer is surprised by their reaction or any ongoing distress. For some officers, what they want or need most is to go back to work taking calls. I recall one officer describing how he wanted to stop thinking and just work.

The supervisor might use her best judgment and decide to assert her authority by assigning impacted officers some alternative duty until the end of the tour or encourage them to switch into their civilian clothes while they write their reports. Permitting an officer to go home early may be an option; however, it should not be assumed that it is preferred. One cop may want to go home and hug his kids, while another lives alone and going home to an empty house may not be helpful. Following psychological trauma, keeping activities close to normal and recognizing that officers may want to be together is important.

Agency Response To Critical Incidents

Sometimes the lasting trauma is not from the event itself, but rather results from how the officer is treated following the event. In order to make this information useful to agencies big and small, I will describe some general concepts that are both scalable and adaptable, as well as some specific processes we follow at my agency of about 600 sworn officers.

Response at Headquarters

I meet privately with each officer designated as having been directly involved in a critical incident before they leave for the day or night. The purpose and function of this meeting is to have a conversation about the potential for, and normalcy of, psychological distress. But more importantly, I want to reassure them they will be fine and introduce the EAP activities in the days to follow. Our conversation is not privileged, as it is when they meet with their attorney, and to protect their interests, we do not speak about the incident. Most often it is hours post-incident, and I am the last to see the officer before they are released to go home. Only on occasion do I find them to be noticeably upset or still feeling the effects of adrenalin or not thinking in their forebrain.

I greet the officer with a calm and friendly face. I shake their hand, as I am genuinely glad to see them. I make no assumption that the officer is harmed, nor am I trying to look into their soul for signs of defect (I have been on the other end of that look, and it is unnerving). I keep it calm, friendly, simple, straightforward and unhurried. I believe my job, in part, is to help them get back fully *into* their thinking brain, if they have not already done so. I am aware that sometimes cops take their temperature off of me, so I calm myself before and during our meeting.

Commonly, it has been a long day, and these officers are often tired and ready to go home or elsewhere. I have gathered the basic facts of the case beforehand. I do the following:

- Remind the officer who I am and why I am there.

- Gather basic contact information, including whom the officer lives with and loved ones they may be concerned about because of their involvement in a critical incident.

- Ask about the people the officer considers to be part of their support system. I do this in part because I want to know who they have and also to get them thinking about it.

- Ask if the officer has had any prior critical incidents.

- Explain the mandated EAP-related activities the next few days. I identify any household scheduling conflicts and time preferences, as I am eager to accommodate the officer's needs as best as possible.

- Rather than describing a long list of signs and symptoms of psychological distress, which I find annoying and too suggestive, I may do a little psycho-education. I tell the officer that critical incidents commonly require super focus and can result in a number of sensory distortions or, gaps and crooked lines in our memory which the officer may have experienced or could experience, especially after some sleep. I tell them that not only is this normal, but it can be a sign of a high-functioning brain, not some kind of defect.

- Ask the officer if they have any concerns or questions.

- Give the officer my card and encourage them to call me anytime. Let them know I will check in with them the next day as well as take the lead in scheduling mandated events.

Sometimes we will talk about a significant other. I will ask if she is the type that wants the gory details or if she is one that he will withhold them from, it goes both ways. Either way, I make a point to ask the officer to share my number with a partner or spouse, parent etc. as they all are welcome to contact me. Not only do loved ones need support, but I am convinced that the best way to support an officer in need is to support the supporter. And the officer owes it to their loved ones to resolve any distress that they are experiencing.

I may reiterate that the officer can call me anytime day or night, I might punctuate that by telling them that after an officer-involved shooting I awoke after a few hours of hard sleep and started to feel crazy as I struggled with the gaps and crooked lines. I wished that I had someone to call to calm me down and help get my mind right. For this officer, that person could be me, or anyone else they trust. Lastly, I thank them for the work they did and depending on the circumstance, remind them that this is what society asks them to do on its behalf.

Days Following and On-going

My agency mandates therapeutic appointments and a group debriefing for officers designated to have been directly involved in critical incidents. They are required to meet one-on-one with a therapist within days of the incident and attend a group debriefing. Later they attend two follow-up sessions with the same therapist, one at three months (90 days) and another at six months (180 days). I schedule and coordinate all these meetings; officers are only required to show up. I also call officers at one year, or on occasion before that if I see fit. In addition to the mandated therapeutic sessions, or check-ins, the officers can request additional services for themselves or their family.

Our agency has not found mandated sessions to be problematic. I make it a priority to accommodate the officers' schedule needs, not mine, and we try to accomplish much of it during their administrative days immediately following the incident. There are different points of view on this, but our agency enjoys many advantages to what has become the expected routine, a new normal. I get little to no resistance to the mandates. I start "selling" it (softening them up to the idea) on our first meeting, and sometimes beforehand in roll call or in-service training. In fact, the complaint sometimes is that we did not mandate enough people.

One of the benefits of mandating debriefing attendance is that all those designated as having been directly involved in a critical incident are in attendance. No one is required to talk, but most do. As is sometimes the case, a senior officer objects saying they were not impacted, but when I explain that their presence may be needed for junior officers, they agree. Also, the invitation includes an acknowledgement that there is no assumption they have been harmed, cannot handle what happened and have not dealt with worse things, but instead emphasizes that we are supporting a system and process of support and speedy recovery. I remind cops that we know they can endure difficulty, but this may not be the time to endure.

Talking about traumas, just forming the words and saying it out loud to a trusted other, can be very liberating. When we gather and share experiences we can fill in gaps and straighten crooked lines in our memory. When a narrative makes sense to us, consistent with what we experienced, our brain can relax, so to speak, stop searching to fill a void, and more easily file it away. We can get relief and be comforted by identifying common themes.

Another thing to consider is that your participation in a therapeutic process can be reassuring to your loved ones. When my wife explained to my youngest child, telling him that I would not be coming home from work right away because I had been involved in a shooting at work, he asked, "Is Dad okay?" She said yes and added, "If Dad felt bad, the people at work would help him." He shrugged contently, saying, "If Dad's okay, I'm okay."

Because I am a sergeant, and most often the people involved in critical incidents are officer rank, I may ask one of my peer support team members to follow-up with select officers, to reach out to them as they see fit. For officer-involved shootings, I call upon one of a group of officers (peer support team members or not) who have also been involved in officer-involved shootings to also check-in with them or act as a buddy of sorts for the weeks and months to come. I have a couple of senior officers that are perfectly suited for this. (Note: Some officers are advised by their attorney to not to speak to anyone about the incident, which could include CISM debriefings.)

Do the Most for the Most

Doing the most for the most can include not trying to do everything for everybody. It is important to find a balance between too much and too little following critical incidents and potentially traumatic events. Cops have told me:

"Debriefs should involve all officers involved in the incident, not just the main people involved."

"I personally did not need to talk to a therapist after my critical incident, but I understand why this is needed."

"It created more stress than anything else."

Cops are rightly suspicious creatures, and I am willing to risk under-achieving to protect the reputation of the process rather than risk overstepping or being too eager to help. I try to maintain a healthy and sustainable balance. I rely on what I learned in ambulance work — the importance of triage. In ambulance work, when attending to just one patient, no matter how sick or injured they were, we could handle it. But with multiple patients, two, three or twenty, things get tricky, and if you fail to triage and try to work miracles with a hopeless or distracting case, another will quietly bleed to death for lack of attention. Assume you do not have unlimited resources, a useful triage philosophy is to *do the most for the most*. Get to the people that need the most (make an educated guess) and hope that everyone else can manage on their own or will ask for help as needed, or attend to them later, or in some cases not at all. Trying to eliminate all potential psychological harm or fix everyone when harm occurs is not only foolhardy but can undermine individual and group processes that have evolved in our police culture to help each other.

Some critical incidents or traumatic events involve huge numbers of officers, a psychological mass casualty of sorts. Even with relatively small events, some individuals will be very impacted, some not at all, most some-where in between. Some of those impacted may not even have been on scene. Unlike physical trauma, psychological trauma is hidden in the head, heart or gut, and will not be obvious like blood on a shirt.

The only way I know how to navigate this on a daily basis is to do the most for the most and not try to do everything for everybody. Additionally, those in a helper role, such as peer support, may need to conserve some energy. It does not help the situation if you crash your squad en route to an *officer needs help* call or as in a foot pursuit, fail to reserve some energy for when you catch the guy in case he fights.

I am eager to help any cop who needs help; I just do not magically know who they are. EAP works best when officers use it as a resource and voluntarily initiate contact because of their confidence in its usefulness and trustworthiness.

Critical Incident Stress Management (CISM)

A CISM team consists largely of public safety people and mental health professionals who volunteer to assist an agency by providing brief group interventions to mitigate the stressors associated with exposure to a critical incidents or potentially traumatic events. These interventions have been formalized into a number of processes depending on the perceived need or situation. It is important to know that although a well-done debriefing can be very helpful, it is only one part of a series of supportive processes.

I would refer the readers to the work of Jeffery Mitchell and the International Critical Incident Stress Foundation (ICISF) and their publication, *Critical Incident Stress Management (CISM): A Practical Review*[14] Included are the core concepts, interventions tactics, and research on CISM, as well as guides for interactive group crisis intervention such as Rest Information Transition Series (RITS), Crisis Management Briefings (CMB), and critical incidents stress diffusings and debriefings.

Some people and organizations have considerable experience in CISM and feel strongly about specific routines and regimens when conducting such things as debriefings. This can be important because these interventions are not without risk and done poorly can cause harm both to the participants and the reputation of the process.

How we approach an officer, or a group of officers, following a critical incident can be a matter of style and is both an art and a science. Your reputation and relationship with officers beforehand is important, which can be enhanced by pre-event education. Word of mouth supporting the benefits and trustworthiness of EAP and CISM interventions are your greatest assets.

Group Debriefings. For cops, gathering informally as a small group and expressing anger, dismay or dark humor are in effect reassuring each other that they are okay and have in fact witnessed the same bad sights and sounds. Just being in the presence of another is comforting and contributes to healing. Humans verbalize thoughts to make sense of their experience or vent emotions. Talking seems to help harmonize both sides of the brain. I have observed that the more coherent the story gets, it seems to be an indication that they are also feeling better. Amongst people you trust, verbalizing thoughts and expressing fears, doubts, and painful memories without being judged can be very helpful, and those listening can benefit as well. A debriefing should be a safe, calm environment where those involved in the event gather and talk about the experience and aftermath. While expressions of strong emotion may occur, we do not seek it as a sign of success and should actively avoid re-traumatizing or attempts to "relive" the event.

We should not assume that those who express strong emotion following a critical incident, traumatic event, or workplace tragedy such as an officer suicide, were more affected or somehow cared more than those who do not. It is probably better to assume that we do not know how others are impacted, and further inquiry may be only partially useful. Thus, it is important to do what can be done, such as provide pre-event education about psychological distress and build post-event systems and processes to mitigate harm and be responsive to requests for help or signs of trouble.

Goals of Debriefing

- Support the process of gathering, talking and listening to each other after a critical incident

- Regain confidence if needed

- Enhance skills to manage mental and physical reactions

- Increase awareness of resources and additional support

Confidentiality. Participants must promise not to talk about what is said in the debriefing with anyone not at the debriefing. If anyone believes they should not speak about something, they should not. Debriefings should not be assumed to be a privileged conversation.

The process of a group debriefing can reveal common themes of psychological or emotional distress such as being surprised, feelings of being unprepared or powerless to prevent or fix something bad, and help-lessness. Just the discovery of this can be helpful.

Therapeutic Response To Critical Incidents and Traumatic Events

Beyond the mandated therapy session already described, additional therapeutic help can be necessary if symptoms are prolonged or problematic. Indicators that an event may have been more impactful are such things as sleep problems, lack of motivation, social withdrawal, anger, intrusive or unwanted images, numbing or mental fog, physical aches and pains, intestinal distress or even teeth clenching. These are not necessarily abnormal responses or unexpected, and it is very reasonable to expect that certain events may leave cops feeling not themselves for a while; however, some psychological trauma does not get better with time. If distress is intense, prolonged, or goes beyond what the officer believes is just feeling bad for a while, they may need further evaluation.

There are different kinds of stress and psychological trauma, as well as different states of mind and wellbeing when they occur. Not all stress is the same and not all traumas are the same, not all people are the same. As cops, if it is cold out we feel cold, raining, wet. If we witness bad things, we may feel bad. **Post traumatic stress (PTS)** is the expected *dis-stress* that may follow traumatic events. Post traumatic stress is a non-diagnostic term, purposely vague, PTSD without the "D" for disorder. If we do not recover, meaning that it persists, or interferes with normal functioning, then it may become a disorder. The word disorder means *out of order,* not broken, but it is an indication that the officer may need professional help to fully recover.

Historically, people may have tried fitting all psychological trauma or extreme stress into a term like "shock". Today we have an expanding list of disorders. The following categories can be useful in helping us understand what might be going on in ourselves or others.

Stress Response to Trauma

The Trauma Dissociation website describes some of the diagnosable and treatable post-traumatic stress responses. The responses include:

- Acute Stress Disorder (ASD) / Acute Stress Reaction
- Adjustment Disorder (AD)
- Posttraumatic Stress Disorder (PTSD)

Acute Stress Disorder (ASD) / Acute Stress Reaction. Acute Stress Disorder is a trauma-related mental health condition that lasts at least 3 days. Acute Stress Reaction, is slightly different and results from an "exceptionally stressful life event" or "continuous trauma", and typically lasts between a few hours and a few days. Both Acute Stress Disorder and Acute Stress Reaction have symptoms which are similar to Posttraumatic Stress Disorder.

- Last from 3 days to 1 month
- Many different symptoms, including:
  Intense reactions to trauma reminders or thoughts
  Avoiding trauma reminders, thoughts or discussion
  Sleep problems

Anger or irritability
Negative emotions
On edge or easily started

Stressful events which do not include severe and traumatic components do not lead to Acute Stress Disorder; Adjustment Disorder may be an appropriate diagnosis. If Acute Stress Disorder persists it may lead to a diagnosis of Posttraumatic Stress Disorder.[15]

Adjustment Disorder (AD). Adjustment Disorder is a stress-related disorder which is caused by a specific stressor where symptoms occur within 3 months. Many different symptoms or concerning behaviors can occur and include feeling prolonged hopelessness, sadness, worry and upset, as well as physical symptoms. These distressing symptoms or behaviors will seem out of proportion to the severity or intensity of the stressor and may significantly impair social, work, or other important areas of functioning. Adjustment disorder is different from normal bereavement.

Where ASD follows a traumatic event, AD may follow any stressful or life event requiring significant adjustment and resolves on its own within months or at the end of the stressor.[16]

Posttraumatic Stress Disorder (PTSD). Posttraumatic Stress Disorder is a mental health disorder that is not caused by normal, everyday stress, but instead most commonly from intense fear, horrific or extreme events such as being assaulted or sexual violence. It can occur at any age and left untreated can last a lifetime.

The four primary symptoms of PTSD are:

- Re-experiencing the trauma psychologically, such as with flashbacks and nightmares

- Avoiding reminders of the trauma

- Emotional numbing

- Hyperarousal, such as irritability and constant hypervigilance

Criteria for diagnosis includes:

- Exposure to actual or threatened death or serious injury to self or others

- Intrusion symptoms associated with the traumatic event

- Persistent avoidance of reminders of the traumatic event

- Negative changes in thinking or mood

- Significant changes in arousal or reactivity

The symptoms must last more than 1 month and cause significant distress in social, work or other areas of functioning, and symptoms are not linked to substance use or other medical conditions.[17]

PTSD can be chronic or severe, but it is also treatable. Most people who have experienced a traumatic event will not develop PTSD. But for those who do, PTSD left unrecognized or untreated can be deadly.

Beyond Talk Therapy and the Role of Bilateral Stimulation

Psychological trauma is very much like it sounds, harm to the psyche. But it can go deeper than just the thinking brain. The animal brain of the human is designed to imprint certain experiences with strong emotion to achieve the ultimate goal, immediate physical survival and long-term continuation of the species, simplistically, to push us to either seek or avoid. After a traumatic event, the mind assumes it could happen again and works to connect the experience to related sights, sounds, smells, and strong feelings or physical sensations. Although useful for survival, this can be the source of continuing distress.

Bessel van der Kolk points out the "the impact of trauma is upon the survival or animal part of the brain. That means that our automatic danger signals are disturbed, and we become hyper- or hypo-active: aroused or numbed out. We become like frightened animals. We cannot reason ourselves out of being frightened or upset. Of course, talking can be very helpful in acknowledging the reality about what's happened and how it's affected you, but talking about it doesn't put it behind you because it doesn't go deep enough into the survival brain"[18]

Exploring these traumas and finding the words can be difficult or impossible in some cases. Some have compared the process of trying to explain your distress to files scattered in a heap. When you finally get around to cleaning things up and put things in order, some of the files cannot be found or are unlabeled, others mislabeled. Since psychological trauma can involve the animal brain, the experience can be below consciousness and non-verbal. More traditional talk therapy can be like talking to an animal, unable to get at these unprocessed or inadequately processed memories.

Memory is not like a firm object, it is malleable. Like something that changes a little or a lot every time you pick it up and look at it, it has become something different when you set it down again. Activating a memory renders it unstable, the images and emotions are susceptible to being changed or purposely altered. Emotional memories automatically undergo change when they are recalled, a process known as reconsolidation.

A particular officer involved in a critical incident could go to a mandated therapy session with a licensed therapist (a one-on-one meeting for them to check in about any concerns or distress). Additionally, they could participate in a group debriefing (the group process where participants expressed some of their thoughts and feelings). Yet, this officer may have lingering distress that the group process or talk therapy did not address. Or maybe their distress is not the result of a recent critical incident but instead they are bothered by an event or events from the more distant past. Eye Movement Integrated therapies or Bilateral Stimulation, could be helpful.

Bilateral Stimulation therapies address the strong emotion, memory and associated trigger connections that result from psychological trauma, as well as treat other conditions. The techniques include **Eye Movement Desensitization and Reprocessing (EMDR) and Accelerated Resolution Therapy (ART)**. These psychological procedures facilitate reprocessing most commonly by use of guided lateral eye movement. Typically, the client sits across from the practitioner who moves her hand back and forth; the client follows with his eyes while imagining the distressing event as instructed. This eye movement, similar to that which occurs during REM sleep, is thought to facilitate a connection between the left and right sides of the brain. The procedure liberates the memory for proper processing, taking advantage of memory reconsolidation. The mind heals itself.

With Bilateral Stimulation techniques, the memories (facts about the trauma) remain, but not the intense original painful emotions or physical responses to them. People may worry they will not feel anything after these treatments, but that is not the case. These techniques lower the intensity of the emotion connected to the memory. Sometimes it is valuable to have emotion with lower intensity connected to the memory. EMDR and ART can complete in hours a process that could otherwise take a lifetime, or not happen at all.

Eye Movement Desensitization and Reprocessing (EMDR). EMDR is "a structured therapy that encourages the patient to briefly focus on the trauma memory while simultaneously experiencing bilateral stimulation (typically eye movements), which is associated with a reduction in the vividness and emotion associated with the trauma memories."[19] Further, "Unlike other treatments that focus on directly altering the emotions, thoughts and responses resulting from traumatic experiences, EMDR therapy focuses directly on the memory, and is intended to change the way the memory is stored in the brain, thus reducing and eliminating the problematic symptoms and facilitates learning."[20]

According Francine Shapiro, developer of EMDR and author of *Eye Movement Desensitization and Reprocessing (EMDR) Therapy*, EMDR is used to:

- Help clients learn from the negative experiences of the past

- Desensitize present triggers that are inappropriately distressing

- Incorporate templates for appropriate future action that allow the client to excel individually and within her/his interpersonal system.[21]

Accelerated Resolution Therapy (ART). Accelerated Resolution Therapy is a form of psychotherapy with roots in existing evidence-based therapies but shown to achieve benefits much more rapidly (usually within 1–5 sessions). Clients who are survivors of sexual abuse or suffer with depression, anxiety, panic attacks, PTSD, substance abuse, and many other mental and physical conditions can experience remarkable benefits starting in the first session. ART is not hypnosis.[22]

The client is always in control of the entire ART session, with the therapist guiding the process. Although some traumatic experiences such as rape, combat experiences, or loss of a loved one can be very painful to think about or visualize, the therapy rapidly moves clients beyond the place where they are stuck in these experiences toward growth and positive changes. The process is very straightforward, using relaxing eye movements and a technique called Voluntary Memory/Image Replacement to change the way in which the negative images are stored in the brain. The treatment is grounded in well-established psychotherapy techniques, and the end result is that traumas and difficult life experiences will no longer trigger strong emotions or physical reactions. Importantly, clients do not even have to talk about their traumas or difficult experiences with the therapist to achieve recovery.[23]

Laney Rosenzweig, the developer of ART, is eager to point out how effective the treatment is in helping police officers feel reset to their original pre-trauma state. She states, "you can change the images, you can change the sensations, and you can remove the symptoms with ART, and you are in control."[24]

EMDR and ART seem to be effective in just a few sessions, whether the client suffers from multiple psychological traumas or a single one, one from the distant past or more recent. These therapies can be particularly attractive to officers and agencies because they can require little or no talking. Possibly the most effective recruiting tool is word of mouth, and the results of EMDR/ART can be impressive. I knew a long-time police therapist who told me, "If I could offer one thing to all police officers, it would be EMDR treatment." An ART practitioner told me that "The worse, or more stubborn the symptoms, the more dramatic the results. And you don't have to talk about it!"

Demonstrations of both EMDR and ART can be viewed online by searching either Accelerated Resolution Therapy or EMDR. (Note: At the time of this writing it is unclear to me how to resolve any perceived conflict regarding EMDR and ART treatment prior to legal testimony.)

Peer Support

Critical incidents will not go unnoticed at most agencies, but potentially traumatic events are mostly open-ended, individualized and can easily go unrecognized. A method or system to "capture" and respond to them may require a number of grassroots efforts or systems that include educating both officers, supervisors and command staff.

Peer support team members can play an important role in coming to the aid of officers following potential traumatic events. Just being a member of the team gives them leeway to start a conversation about the mental and emotional impact of bad calls. At my agency, we have a process where if the EAP or a peer support team member is made aware of a potentially traumatic event, we will contact the officer or officers involved. It is simply a personal contact, usually a phone call to check-in with them. Peer support will be covered more fully in Chapter 10 and includes a detailed guide for this check-in.

The Importance of Rest and Recovery: Too Much or Too Soon

Too much psychological trauma could be the flash-bang of a single intense, dramatic or deeply personal event. Too much can also take the form of too soon, a second event when your defenses are down, so to speak, or more like a slow burn, what we might think of as an accumulation of psychological traumas. Whether the trauma you experience resembles more of a flash bang or slow burn, health and wellbeing depend on recovery. A point of view that recognizes the role of restoration in mitigating harm can also be reassuring to officers who fear they have experienced too much bad stuff. I know some officers worry that they are becoming ticking time bombs, and they may suddenly snap. The view of a hidden disease waiting within, sounds mysterious and sinister, and could cause officers undue concern. Possibly more accurate and reassuring is the view that with rest, recovery and if needed, treatments specifically well-suited for psychological trauma, they can be free of such concerns.

CHAPTER 6

GENERAL MENTAL AND EMOTIONAL DISTRESS

Slow Burn

Pigs are Tough

I knew a guy with a pig, a pet pig. The pig had a bad leg as a result of an untreated injury from years earlier when the pig leapt out of a car window on a turn; the pig hated car rides. Years later when the pig finally died after what the owner thought was a short illness, he felt bad when he learned from the veterinarian that the pig had likely been suffering a long time. The vet consoled him with the insight that pigs are good at suffering, enduring and thus hiding their decline. There was help for the sick pig, and the longtime owner would have been glad to provide it had he only known, or the pig would have asked for help, but pigs are tough.

Cops are good at suffering, and even if they wanted sympathy, to whom can they complain, another cop? They are accustomed to physical discomfort, so much about our job can be uncomfortable, even the clothing and equipment we wear as part of our uniform. Imagine this, a battle-ready medieval knight taking a burglary report while wearing a suit of armor, "Ma'am, did you leave the moat's drawbridge down?" We even hang a 3-ounce metal badge on our shirt. Additionally, a police officer's body may hurt from old injuries; we have been in squad wrecks, fights and falls. Tolerating physical discomfort may translate to doing the same for mental and emotional distress.

We might think of this hidden suffering as mental toughness, a necessary element of police work. Much of what needs to be learned in police work must come from direct experience, and some of it comes the hard way. We are proud of our mental toughness and for good reason. Our work descends from a long line of brave men and women who go into the unknown, despite dangers or difficulty.

But this attitude may come at a cost, and when an officer finally declines so significantly that he gets noticed in the form of a work or personal life crisis, it may seem easy in hindsight to say, "Why didn't he get help?" But we do not know what we do not know, and sometimes the decline is slow, strongly encouraged by our surroundings, or involves any number of personal factors. Oftentimes we do not know better or are not ready for a message saying otherwise. Before we use this as evidence that we are powerless victims of our career, we must see our part in it.

Neglect or inattention to our wellbeing as police officers can be due to issues of identity and distraction as discussed in Chapter 1. If we take better care of ourselves, maybe the harmful exposures that slip past our armor or those that otherwise seem to exceed our ability to cope would be better managed.

Shadow Resume

All of us have a shadow resume which we may not talk about, the tough things we have faced, whether as a child or adult, that effect how we live our life and survive physically and socially. How we manage the stresses of police work has a lot, if not all, to do with what we bring to the job, not only from our upbringing, but also from how much rest we got the day or night before our shift. Also, what we dislike about the job might have nothing to do with the job; it is just a convenient target.

Police officers value their route to mental toughness, and though it serves us well at times, we pay a price for it. The long list of the signs and symptoms from repeated exposure to stress and psychological trauma can look both concerning and familiar, and include feeling hypervigilant or hopeless, helpless and sleepless.

It is up to the officer to decide what is too much. And cops should consider that they tend to endure more mental and emotional pain and suffering than necessary. I think I know why. It is in part because cops are tough, we are proud of that, we do good, necessary, hard work. But police officers also think they are supposed to suffer more, and maybe within limits this is true in the sense that we are strong and protect the weak, we can endure.

Something else to consider, however, is that we have all turned down, muted or become deaf to our alarm systems. We may only casually notice things that would alarm "normal" people. I once heard a cop say, "When I talk with other cops I feel normal and healthy, but when I talk with non-cops, I sometimes think maybe there is something wrong with me." We do these unnatural things that are dramatic such as running toward gunshots, but we routinely do less dramatic things like walk into a dark alley at night looking for trouble. In order to do these things, we must turn down the alarms, the impulses to not do them. These muted alarms allow us to do our work but can cause problems for us because we may also ignore vague discomfort or worry and wait too long before we see trouble within, letting too much damage occur before we act. And it is a damn shame, because when cops wait too long, suffer too much, it not only harms them, but their relationships as well. That too may not seem so dramatic at first, such as when we are mentally absent, not fully present, or lack full engagement in our lives, but our loved ones suffer, they do not get our best.

Officer Needs Help, the subtitle of Chapter 7, suggests an urgent call where everyone stops what they are doing and races to the cop's aid. These are thankfully rare. Urgent calls for help from the public, true 911 emergencies, are a sudden event, but even those can often be traced back to a slow burn, gradual decline, neglect of some sort, inattention, or people putting themselves in dangerous positions. Cops can neglect things too; they can be so busy showing up at other people's shit shows that they may not notice their own.

The help cops need is more like the broken window, little signs of disorder that are significant. The Broken Window criminology theory can be applied to ourselves. We need to take better care of ourselves, to see trouble early. We need to be tough, but not as tough as the tough world we police.[1] We can act tough when we are out there exchanging hard looks with a bad guy, but we must also maintain our soft side and possibly our greatest advantage for health and wellbeing, our loving family at home. If we have suffered too much harm or our memories cause us to painfully re-experience the emotion of an event, then it may be useful to seek good expert help.

Know Better

Amongst public safety workers, we tend to focus on critical incidents and traumatic events as our greatest source of harm. This is due in part to the fact that these are easier to identify and talk about because they are often sudden and dramatic. There is often little to no shame or stigma when dealing with a critical incident compared to struggles with depression or substance abuse. Yet, general mental and emotional distress is more common, probably causes the most distress, and along with behavioral health crises, requires far more mental health resources than critical incidents do.

Because some agencies appropriately want to do more for officers mental and emotional wellbeing, and sometimes they are compelled to do more, they must know better. The subject of officer mental and emotional distress can be difficult for a number of reasons. The subject is complex, and the topic itself may make us uncomfortable as we reflect on our own mental health struggles. As officers, talking about what often translates to "feelings" may be both unpracticed and risky, as it may contradict a view of strength and self-reliance. There is a strong impulse to avoid difficult things and to keep what might feel shameful hidden as we cannot help but compare how we are feeling on the inside to how others appear on the outside.

We have successfully raised the expectation of wellbeing around physical health and fitness. We should also raise the expectation for mental health and wellbeing. Another benefit of promoting wellness generally, or specifically around certain skills such as healthy thinking, is that not all staff need to hear the message for all staff to benefit. When individuals become aware of their own or others negative thinking, it makes going back to old unhealthy ways of thinking and behaving more difficult or in some cases impossible. For example, dispelling the myth of a "functional alcoholic" (unless that definition is they have not gotten fired or died yet) makes believing that myth again impossible. When a certain critical mass of people within a group start to think and behave in a healthy way, it makes expressions of poor thinking and behaving more conspicuous, more obvious, the bad behavior stands out.

If we know better, we can do better. Openly discussing behavioral health issues may not feel natural and may be extremely difficult, but it becomes easier with practice. The subject of alcohol misuse is a good example. For every cop who rejects or pushes against bringing up the problem, there is a cop who asks why it took so long to talk openly about a common problem.

It is unhelpful to be too eager to diagnose yourself or others with mental health problems for a variety of reasons, including that we may not know what we are talking about. Additionally, some problems overlap or are co-occurring, meaning more than one condition exists at the same time. Also, these are just categories, an attempt to organize the essentially un-organizable human psyche. The complexity of humans can be better appreciated with a basic understanding of different types of mental health problems, disorders, difficult feelings and behaviors.

General Mental and Emotional Distress

General mental and emotional distress is the range of psychological problems that all humans may suffer. These are not law enforcement specific or unique to police work or necessarily occur because of the work. They could be related to the job, but more likely, struggles here have to do with your genetics, how healthfully you were raised, and how you cope with the mental and emotional distressing parts of the job and life.

The large category of mental and emotional distress can be broken down into a number of subtopics, for example, sleep problems, anxiety or financial concerns. Each may be viewed separately with a unique remedy. Commonly however, psychological issues are interrelated, or co-occurring, such as when a sleep problem is related to psychological trauma or anxiety is related to substance misuse. Examples of general mental and emotional distress include the following:

- Anxiety and depression

- Family and relationship conflicts

- Sleep problems

- Loss and grief

- Work stress and frustration

- Injury, illness and chronic pain

- Substance misuse

- Financial and legal concerns.

These are problems all humans struggle with. In the arch of a career or a lifetime, a cop is going to experience some or all of them. In my job as EAP director, over 90% of the demand for services are voluntary requests and the vast majority are for things from this list.

Each of these examples have specific treatment plans and solutions. I will not address all of these issues separately, however anxiety and depression are so common that I will cover them later in the chapter. There are any number of resources for each of these topic areas, including self-help books, health insurance provider offerings, or qualified professional help. The desire and motivation to seek help often precedes locating the resource. This is why even without individual requests for help, health education initiatives can bring these issues into everyone's awareness.

From my experience working with officers, I have found that three primary factors contribute to their general mental and emotional distress:

- Nature or nurture influences

- Little "t" psychological trauma

- Adaptive and maladaptive law enforcement career coping.

Nature or Nurture

The word nature in this context refers to what people are born with and includes propensities toward certain illnesses or problems. Therapists sometimes refer to this as a client having to fight their biology, whether it is weight loss, substance misuse, depression, anxiety or whatever. The nurture part is how you were loved and cared for as a child.

Most everyone has something from their family of origin that left a mark on them, setting them up for certain issues or problems that eventually need addressing as an adult. In other words, what it took to survive childhood and adolescence may have left us with some slight or extremely unhealthy attitudes, beliefs or behaviors that are no longer necessary or useful as adults, yet people continue to hold on to them. These unhealthy habits are especially likely to come out when we have low mood, low self-esteem or feel anxious. Some people may be completely unaware of the link between their "issues" and nature-nurture factors. Maturing requires that we undo or unlearn some of our mistaken beliefs and childhood adaptations that we no longer need.

Not all childhoods are equal, and some are much more difficult than others. Adverse childhood experiences, as defined by the ACE study, are a great disadvantage. The Center for Disease Control and Prevention-Kaiser Permanente's Adverse Childhood Experiences (ACE) study found that psychological trauma experienced by children leads to all kinds of trouble later in life including: social, emotional and cognitive impairment; adoption of health-risk behavior; social problems; disease, disability and even early death.[2] The experience of danger, for example, produces a stress response that can be preserved as part of an amazing design to protect us in case it happens again. The problem is this built in warning system that can be lifesaving, can also be health damaging. Likely, much of police work is dealing with the aberrant behavior of those who have suffered mental and emotional harm as children. Interestingly, some cops' own adverse childhood experiences may have drawn them into the career in the first place.

We all must deal with the bodies we were born with and the lives we were born into. Despite seemingly huge setbacks or disadvantages, some people not only survive, but thrive, whereas some hugely advantaged people appear to make little life progress or seem to decline or squander opportunity. This may speak to a third ingredient, one that can be learned — stick-to-itiveness, the ability to overcome or persevere.

Little "t" Psychological Trauma

As covered in Chapter 5, not all psychological trauma is the same. In police work, little "t" trauma is much more common, but less dramatic and possibly, over time, more harmful. It can be like a slow burn, a gradual decline. It is difficult to know when it started, or how it is related or unrelated to other events in your life. Many cops eagerly describe psychological trauma as cumulative.

Although it may feel cumulative, I am not sure this is so. It may be more accurate and useful to view the lingering effects of psychological trauma as poor or incomplete recovery from the last trauma, like burning a sunburn, a lack of healing from the previous wound. It is very possible that the little "t" traumas are the most harmful for officers. What feels like accumulation might be a decreased willingness or ability to tolerate additional psychological trauma, where a little can easily become too much. The sunburn analogy emphasizes rest and recovery, time away from the job, or figuratively, out of the sun. Humans are remarkably well equipped to recover from hardships; otherwise we would not have survived as a species. But we want to do more than just survive, and this requires going beyond our evolutionary impulses.

Adaptive and Maladaptive Law Enforcement Career Coping

Police work can be a very seductive career, one with lots of interesting, exciting, alluring sights, sounds, and experiences. The rules of life bend, as you become prince of the city. Combine this with a ready-made identity; an officer may remain distracted from the necessary work of maturation and personal growth year after year. Some signs of trouble can be subtle such as less joy, as when you notice you do not take as much pleasure in the things you previously enjoyed. Or you experience increased isolation. In a sense, your world becomes smaller. Not so subtle things could be increased anger. This can find easy expression on the job, or it might reveal itself at home. I have had cops say to me, "My kids are afraid of me." Or, "My wife says that

I'm pissed off all the time." Anger is not all bad, but it can be an indicator of unprocessed emotions. No matter what the source, anger problems can be a great starting point for self-reflection and/or therapeutic help.

How do humans respond to trouble or difficulties? They adapt one way or another. Adaptation can take three forms:

- Healthy adaptation

- Problematic adaptation

- Unhealthy adaptation or maladaptation.

An example of healthy adaptation could be a callus on your hand, your skin thickening in the exact spot where it gets the most wear and tear. A healthy adaptation for a cop could be developing thick skin metaphorically, being less sensitive and more impervious to hostility. Problematic adaptation could be a necessary adaptation, but one that causes other problems, such as police cynicism or being perceived as insensitive due to thick skin. *Mal* means faulty or bad. Maladaptation is a response that is more harmful than helpful, and is seen in any number of behavioral health crises.

Adaptive coping includes such things as some amount of healthy cynicism, maladaptive coping takes it to an extreme, allowing cynicism to dominate your worldview. Often maladaptive coping includes avoidance or compounding an issue in such a way as to undermine health. We can think of examples at our agency of people who have managed to cope very well. They are the ones who are helpful and supportive of their coworkers; they are productive and constantly contribute at work while having a rich personal life. And we know very well, the people who are not coping well. Coping, well or not, is an individual responsibility; however, coworkers, supervisors, and leaders in an organization may be able to help. This includes raising the expectation of wellbeing.

An officer's sense of purpose and function may stay consistent throughout her career or evolve as she or the job changes. Many experienced cops can relate to an early period when the work gladly consumed them. Then a period of disillusionment followed, from which they eventually emerged either with a better practice of balance and a renewed sense of purpose, or as dispirited, entrenched in anger and counting their time until retirement.

I avoid using the word *burnout* because I think it suggests that a workers' actions were so virtuous and required so much self-sacrifice that burnout was inevitable. In reality, for some it probably means they either overinvested or underinvested in the work. Others did not have the right temperament for the work in the first place or simply did not effectively adapt. I have noticed that for every so-called rotten job that exists, there is someone who loves doing that "rotten" job. People who really like or love their job do not get "burned out." For many people who do get burned out, they are, as the title of Herbert Freudenberger's classic book on the subject states, paying the *high cost of high achievement*. So-called burnout can be a natural consequence for some workers as they try to be high achievers or experience disillusionment or disappointment regarding their expectations about the work.

A reasonable goal might be to increase healthy adaptation, manage problematic adaptation, and get help with maladaptation.

Anxiety and Depression

For many, general mental and emotional distress is synonymous with anxiety and depression. Mild anxiety and depression may be a necessary response to grief, loss, and transition. A simplistic view might be that anxiety is a type of fear while depression is more of a shutting down or a defense against some other emotion. A certain amount of anxiety, and maybe depression, may be the cost of being human with a large thinking brain, the "dizziness of freedom."[3]

Anxiety and depression are very common, sometimes recognized as such, sometimes not. People visit the doctor for a variety of reasons; however, it is not uncommon that the primary reason or underlying cause is actually a mental health issue. Anxiety and depression have been described as the *common colds of mental illness;* largely because they are so prevalent. There are different types of anxiety and depression all of which affect how you feel, think and behave to varying degrees, and range from mild to severe. But unlike a cold, you do not catch depression. Physicians and therapists have suggested a better metaphor is to compare depression to diabetes. Both are diseases of modern life, need to be managed behaviorally, and possibly with medication, while requiring self-monitoring and self-care. Beyond metaphors, anxiety and depression should each be recognized as being both diseases of their own[4] and related to the health of society or the community in which someone lives.

Anxiety can feel like a nagging unease or persistent fear coloring your view of everything. Some people experience panic attacks where they feel overwhelmed by frightening thoughts and sensations. Most people experience anxiety as mild and only occasionally related to specific events or concerns. However, some people experience more frequent or intense symptoms that may be diagnosed as an anxiety disorder. Anxiety (including panic attacks) is treatable with cognitive behavioral therapy, sometimes medication, calming techniques and other self-care.

Those suffering persistent depression or anxiety for example not only struggle with a number of issues, but it can put them at a social disadvantage as well, and easily lead to isolation and shame, probably the exact opposite of what they need most. It is useful for the rest of us to understand this, so we can recognize those who are suffering and at the very least not add to their burden. If you ask a clinician for a list of signs and symptoms of depression, she will provide a list that is quite forgettable and unhelpful to us as individuals or cops. But if you ask someone who actually suffers from depression you will get a different list. This list of "25 'Embarrassing' Symptoms of Depression We Don't Talk About"[5] was created by an online blog community supporting people struggling with depression. The list was collected from those who suffer depression, and I believe you will find it memorable.

- Not showering
- Avoiding loved ones
- Digestive issues
- Wasting time
- Taking frequent naps
- Loneliness
- Low confidence
- Matted hair and bed sores
- Poor concentration
- Feeling like a bad parent
- Dissociation
- Being unable to leave the house
- Feeling emotional "extremes"
- Low sex drive
- Not cleaning
- Lack of dental hygiene
- Oversleeping
- "Flaking" on plans
- Not knowing when you'll cry next
- Brain fog
- Weight change
- Feeling tired all the time
- Not being able to work fulltime
- Feeling angry
- Compulsive skin picking

In some cases, anxiety and depression can be closely related to each other with areas of overlap without distinct borders. In other cases, they are distinctly different and unrelated. Some anxiety and especially depression can be so extreme as to be debilitating and life-threatening. It is not within the scope of this book to speak at length about this or other psychiatric disorders, illnesses or diseases, other than to comment briefly about medication use by police officers and the topic of officer suicide prevention. It is very important that those who suffer from anxiety or depression seek medical evaluation, medication as needed, self-help books, talk therapy, Cognitive Behavioral Therapy (CBT), EMDR/ART, as well as learn new skills to manage worry and negative self-talk.

Expert medical and psychological care, which may include medications, helps people manage anxiety and depression. Individuals should also simultaneously manage their sleep, avoid drugs and alcohol, treat physical illnesses, eat well, and stay physically and socially active.

Antianxiety medication and antidepressants. Anxiety and depression are treatable via a variety of means, including psychoactive medication. Whether it is a chief of police or a patrol officer who is prescribed the medication, it is important for not only them but also for society that the medication be taken as needed. Taking antidepressants or antianxiety drugs does not keep you from being a cop.

Finding the right medication and dose can be complex and takes time. *Psychologists* or therapists cannot prescribe medications. Your general medical doctor can prescribe medication. *Psychiatrists* are medical doctors who specialize in psychiatry. They can prescribe psychoactive medications and they have the expertise to do the necessary adjustments and follow-up. However, first appointments with a psychiatrist can take weeks to months. This is why you are often advised to see your general medical doctor first.

Cops can be misdiagnosed and ineffectively or even inappropriately medicated if the clinician is not skilled and unfamiliar with psychological trauma, chronic stress and some of the personality traits of police officers. Rather than making cops and their loved ones reluctant to get help, these concerns should make them cautious and inquisitive about treatments. Unmanaged, persistent depression is dangerous and the general belief is that the earlier depression is treated, the easier it is to treat.

It is important to take medications as prescribed and follow all recommendations. I have noticed that people frequently fail to take even simple over-the-counter medications, such as ibuprofen, correctly. For example, instead of following the instructions to take the recommended dose every 4–6 hours, someone might gobble down a few and neglect to take more until the pain returns. In order for a medication to achieve and maintain a therapeutic level (meaning sustained effectiveness), they need to be ingested at the recommended interval. Failing to do this causes a see-saw effect, dipping below the therapeutic level as they wear off and in effect requiring a start-over rather than a continuous level so they can work as designed. Any benefit of a medication can be lost due to a lack of compliance with instructions.

Agencies vary on how they regulate medication use. Some have drug policies and random drug testing for the entire staff or certain work groups

(SWAT, bomb squad, negotiators). Prohibited drugs may include certain prescribed or even over-the-counter medications. Basic screening detects only drugs of abuse for five specific substances: cannabinoids (marijuana/hash), cocaine (cocaine, crack, benzoylecgonine), amphetamines (amphetamines, methamphetamines, speed), opiates (heroin, codeine, opium, morphine), and phencyclidine (PCP). A drug policy may use language similar to this: "any officer who is, via a valid doctor's prescription, using a medication that will, after drug screening, test positive, is required to notify the department human resource unit of said fact."[6]

Officers, who have been appropriately evaluated, prescribed medication and are medically followed by their physicians should take their medication as prescribed without hesitation, and generally, it is nobody's business but yours and your doctor's. It is the physician's duty to inform patients of any potential side effects that could negatively impact or impair the officer's ability to perform their duties, and it is the officer's duty to be alert to them. I once had an officer call and without introduction blurt out, "Do I have to tell work that I take antidepressants?" I replied, "Nope" and he hung up. Officers should take the medications they need to take, and it is not the agency's business unless the officer cannot do his duty or there is a policy describing which medications (prescription or over-the-counter) must be reported. As a society, we want people taking their required medications, whether they are cops, commercial airline pilots, or anyone else.

Tribe Support

Those suffering a hardship can be pleasantly surprised by who and how many people offer support and encouragement; they might have had no idea so many people cared. Where I work we have a full range of people who have suffered terrible tragedies or more common losses. I keep a mental note of officers who have lost a spouse, a child, or suffered a particular hardship or prolonged discipline as just a few examples, to call upon and ask if they would be willing to reach out to another officer with a similar hardship. As tough and hard as cops can be, it is remarkable how much comfort they can provide for each other.

Certainly, some people feel desperately alone in their suffering. They may choose to keep it private or want help but feel too ashamed to ask. Coworkers sometimes fail to recognize their distress and calls for help or do not know how to respond. Formalized Peer Support Teams can meet some of these needs but will never replace the power of having all cops watch out for each other.

It takes courage to reach out to another officer and we can easily talk ourselves out of it, unfortunately we may never know how regrettable that is. That is to say, they were suffering, we noticed something, but failed to act. Likely, a text message is better than just thinking about it, a phone call is better than a text, and face-to-face visit may be better than a phone call.

Effective and Informed Supervision

Supervisory action or intervention in the area of general mental and emotional distress can range from no involvement ("It's none of my business") to direct orders or mandates ("Do your job" or "Get help or get disciplined"). Generally, if an employee satisfactorily meets work expectations, the employer should stay out of their personal life. When an officer's behavior gets a supervisor's attention, the supervisor should first determine if the behavior is related to an unmet work expectation, and next they must decide if some action must be taken.

The employer is responsible to hold employees accountable to work expectations, and the employee is responsible to meet work expectations. In all cases, an informed supervisor will be able to:

1. Recognize serious trouble;

2. Not make things worse by inaction or enabling behavior; and

3. If unsure how to proceed, know where to go for guidance.

Attention to personal health and wellness is every employee's responsibility as they remain fit for duty and contribute to a high-functioning workplace. All police department employees must meet work expectations and seek resolution, intervention, and/or therapeutic treatment for any mental or emotional condition that adversely affects the exercise of their assigned duty.[7] When mental or emotional problems are discovered, supervisors should guide employees toward appropriate resources, which include supervisory coaching, peer support team coaching, EAP resources and personal health insurance plans.

Therapy and the Therapeutic Process

Police agencies or individuals eager to attend to behavioral health needs can seek the services of high-quality professional therapeutic help. Therapy can be a very good way to make mental and emotional progress or speed recovery from distress, but it is not the only way and I respect an officer's suspicions about it. I would like to express some concerns about therapy that may seem contrary to the standard or expected message.

Much of modern psychology places its emphasis on feelings and staying in touch with them. Currently, society further places emphasis on indulging feelings and venting them without reservation. This is in contrast to *conquering* feelings, which some might view disparagingly as equated with stuffing them down. You will recall that I spend some time in chapter 2 emphasizing for cops the importance of letting feelings "have their say," in other words, identifying, and experiencing feelings, in particular the difficult uncomfortable ones. Yet, I am also willing to see some value in what in the past was described as "keeping a stiff upper lip." I say this because modern psychology should not be seen as the answer to all mental and emotional problems, and I am willing to entertain the idea that it could cause some problems. Psychology is a system of knowledge, a way of knowing, but not the only way of knowing and self-improvement.

Police officers seem to be of the *stiff upper lip* type, which must be useful or else they would not have adopted it so readily. So, it seems reasonable to not try to talk cops out of what seems necessary, natural and useful to them, but instead help them see where the therapeutic process has value.

We should be suspicious of our tendency to want to eliminate feeling bad as quickly and painlessly as possible. Depression for example, could be seen as an intruder, where we overreact by either trying to barricade the front door or run out the back door. Instead, we might wrestle with it and on closer examination discover the intruder is actually an old neglected friend with whom we last parted on less than ideal terms. Feeling bad could be an important indicator that some part of our life needs attention. It *is* possible to live wrong. Some depression could be a result of aimlessness or confusion about how we are living, for example, a wise part of ourselves signaling that our values are not right or that we have the right values but are seeking them in the wrong way. And if we are living wrong, how would we know if it were not for mental and emotional distress, and we should welcome that messenger arriving at our door.

So, treating depression could include, seeing a therapist, taking medications if prescribed, and maybe just as importantly, maintaining an orderly and disciplined life — attending daily to what we understand to be our responsibilities or purpose. If your purpose is unclear, consider what you hope to achieve and take the necessary next step. If your path is obstructed, fix the things over which you have control and immediately start to act better.

As best as I can tell, living well requires wisdom, and wisdom is earned the hard way, through pain and suffering of some sort, including mental and emotional distress. Suffering gets our attention and we can respond by one of two paths, becoming more conscious or less conscious. Going into the suffering increases our consciousness, avoiding the distress results in less consciousness, or we may seek "unconsciousness" (for example drinking) to avoid suffering or distress all together. Good therapy can help someone confront or face what he or she is avoiding, not seeing, or fearing most. When I was a field training officer, I was most interested in what a new cop thought was their greatest deficit, their weakest skill, what they feared most, so we could work on that. I based this on what I wished someone would have done for me at a number of stages of my life. What we need most can be what we avoid most.

I recognize some depression can be a dangerous and deadly condition, and I do not wish to minimize it. But I do not want to be paralyzed by that admission and not be able to acknowledge that it can be an understand-able, although very uncomfortable, reaction to difficult circumstances. Thus, I also recognize not ever cop in mental and emotional distress needs therapy, most need courageous self-reflection and good council. This can come in many forms, including therapy. With this caution having been stated, I am now eager to encourage officers to seek high-quality profes-sional help, including therapeutic help as needed.

Good help may require hard work to find and cost some money to obtain. There is a lot of bad advice out there, free and readily available. Short cuts, whether motivated to save money or to avoid pain, can be extremely costly in the long-run. Marriage counseling, treating depression, beginning recovering from a substance use disorder take time and money, but consider the alternative, failure will predictably damage your relation-ships, f-up your kids, get you fired, make you miserable, and cause you to die a slow death. A slow death is a death that for some is starting now.

Help with troubles can come from effective and informed supervision, peer support, agency chaplains, EAP coaching or access to psychological therapy. The last is often provided by people outside of the police culture.

Police officers share with all humans a range of mental and emotional struggles and potential disorders and disease. What all humans do not share with police officers is some of the unique stressors of police work. Unique, even among other public safety workers, in that police officers must be continuously on guard for sudden violence perpetrated by another human wishing to do them harm. The end result is a potential for a health and well-ness decline made more difficult to treat because police officers can become estranged from society leaving officers feeling that they cannot be understood. If mental health professionals do not understand these differences, they risk misdiagnosis, causing harm, or at the very least being ineffective.

Professional Help

Humans are very complex and mental health problems can have a wide range of causes, including our biology, life experiences, and life style. It is important to remember that just because we may not know exactly what causes someone to experience a mental health problem, this does not mean it is any less serious than any other illness, any less deserving of recognition and treatment, or any easier to recover from.[8] What is most important is that you seek help, learn to care for yourself, practice healthy thinking, and know that you are not alone.

Receiving a diagnosis can be a positive experience. You might feel relieved that you can put a name to what is wrong, and it can help you and your doctor discuss what kind of treatment might work best for you. However, a lot of people, including some doctors and psychologists, feel this medical model of diagnosis and treatment is not enough. For example, you might feel the diagnosis you are given does not fully fit your experiences, or that it is simplistic and puts you in a box. Other factors, such as your background, lifestyle and other personal circumstances, may be just as important in understanding what you are experiencing and working out how best to help you feel better. A diagnosis does not have to shape your entire life and may come to be a relatively minor part of your identity.[9] In some situations, a desire to avoid a diagnosis entirely or see a diagnosis as only temporary could be a sign of healthy self-reliance. Others have found it useful to be more selective with the language, for example, avoiding phrases such as "my anxiety" or "my depression," and instead choosing, "the anxiety" and "the depression."

Therapeutic Process

Peer support and coaching can be powerfully effective. But it has its limits and some officers want or need professional psychological help, not necessarily because they are so harmed or damaged, but because they may need what other officers cannot provide, that is, among other things, a point-of-view outside of the police department. Skilled therapists can remind officers of what they share with all humans and guide them more deeply into the therapeutic process.

We can think of the therapeutic process like a pyramid with five levels. At the base is permission, then education, support, counseling and then finally therapy. As the EAP director, I frequently act as a coach, giving officers permission to feel bad or confused about their distress. I actively engage in education about common distressing problems and EAP services, and I support the process for rest and recovery. Therapists do the same but continue in the world of counseling and therapy. The line between support and counseling is not always clear, and we may rightly offer counsel to an officer in distress, but it is otherwise a helpful dividing line. Leave therapy to the professionals. Trained EAP coaches and peer support team members help officers in distress by offering nonjudgmental acceptance, shared experience and support them in the process of self-discovery.

Talk Therapy

Professional therapy can take several forms, and it is probably not far off of what people imagine, talking about your thoughts and feelings. Therapists are well-trained and skilled in listening for certain things and encouraging exploration for the sources of distress. The result can be new ways of thinking and behavior change.

Cognitive Behavioral Therapy (CBT) is a common form of therapy. CBT is a relatively short-term treatment which aims to identify connections between your thoughts, feelings and behaviors, and to help you develop practical skills to manage any negative patterns that may be causing you difficulties.[10] If successful, people learn to recognize and interrupt unhelpful thoughts and change behavior.

Marriage or couples counseling can be enormously helpful and one of the most effective therapeutic processes. Some cops have told me that a single session was transformative. Although therapists may not appreciate this description, marriage counselors can act like a referee, managing a conversation. At home, the emotions sometimes run too hot and you need a neutral third-party to make sure each person is heard. Some cops reach out to me and it seems obvious the damage within their marriage is too great or that they just want out, other times they have been frightened about an intense disagreement. Even for those whose marriage is ending, engaging in a therapeutic process can be very important.

Therapists have told me that their favorite clients are those eager to do the necessary work to get better and "graduate" from therapy. This likely involves some unpeeling of the layers of the past, but that could go on for a long time, and much of it is guess work. So effective therapy can be hard work and involve facing difficult things and learning new skills. Some of the greatest breakthroughs in life come when a friend or acquaintance cares enough, or the therapist is skilled enough to challenge our thinking. Some individuals return to therapy after having taken some time away to address new issues or go deeper into old ones. Certainly, some people have complex histories or multilayered problems, but even they are in charge of their progress and should think critically about it and use therapy for their benefit.

Finding A Therapist

The term mental health professional is a general description for someone who is involved in education or providing behavioral health services. It should not be presumed that a "professional" is skilled at diagnosing or treating mental health disorders. Licensed therapists must achieve and maintain certain standards of the state where they practice, and this can be a good indication of a skilled practitioner. Therapists generally have a master's or doctorate degree. A counselor may or may not have these qualifications. For example, a person may describe themselves as a counselor when their only qualification is that they have spent time in recovery themselves. Seeking help from a licensed therapist is always recommended.

Therapists can be found within your health insurance plan, meaning they are an employee of a particular provider covered under your health insurance. More often, therapists exist in private practice, meaning they run an independent business as a sole proprietor or a small group. They usually charge an hourly or per-session rate and accept cash (private pay) or your health insurance if they are in your network.

Some large police agencies have therapists on staff in the police department. Other agencies, like mine, contract with a number of therapists in private practice who are paid per session by the police department at a negotiated rate. An advantage of an agency paying for therapeutic sessions is that the therapist is not required to render a diagnosis for the purpose of insurance reimbursement.

Note About Fitness For Duty

In order for the therapeutic process to work, officers need to feel that honestly expressing their thoughts and concerns will not be used to evaluate their ability to be a police officer. There are certainly situations where serious problems are discovered, which may concern the officer or therapist and require further evaluation, but the therapeutic session is oriented toward addressing mental and emotional distress and getting better and is not an evaluation of Fitness for Duty. The two do not mix.

A *Fitness for Duty* assessment is an administrative process conducted by a specially qualified therapist or psychiatrist. It is intended to determine if an officer is mentally and physically fit to maintain his police powers. This is evaluative and not therapeutic. The process is a type of forensic psychological evaluation that includes in-person assessment, evaluations and testing, and review of past medical history. It generally requires hours of work and is expensive. It results in a report and recommendation given to the chief or sheriff. Fitness for Duty will be discussed again in Chapter 7.

Vetted Therapists

Therapists for cops need to be carefully selected to find those with the necessary skills, temperament, police cultural competency and attitude about cops. They must be able to handle clients that may have a gun on their hip, and critical colleagues who ask them why they "help the bad guys."

You do not necessarily need a therapist who is an ex-cop and may in fact prefer one without police experience. My most beloved and sought-after therapists have never been cops, and cops can really benefit from learning how the rest of the world views the world. But you do need therapists with some understanding of the work and respect for the worker. What I really like is when a prospective therapist says their brother is a cop, or their favorite uncle was a cop, which means they love a cop. False narratives about police officers are widely accepted, and a therapist who cannot see what is real can harm a vulnerable officer. And an officer who feels unfairly judged by a therapist will make little progress.

What is needed are skilled mental health providers with some understanding of the unique stressors of police work and an appreciation of the heart of a cop. An example of misunderstanding the cop is the belief that the greatest stress comes from working the street, where for many officers, that is the easy part. Instead, it is managing the "politics" of work, home and personal life. Or as Kent Williams puts it, walking not two dogs (balancing work and home life) as most people struggle with, but adding a third dog called the street. Walking three dogs. And the street dog is the easy one for cops. Therapists must also be aware, as Williams points out, a cop's greatest fear is getting caught trusting too much or controlling too little.[11]

It is not helpful if the therapist is traumatized by a cop's storytelling. A cop once told me that he found it very distracting when his therapist winced and shuttered when he relayed what he thought was only mildly gory details about an incident. Therapists working with cops will benefit from an appreciation of how psychological trauma is part of police work. I have noticed that there appear to be more therapists interested in treating psychological trauma. This is an emerging field and some therapists have experience treating soldiers, although the experience may not be perfectly transferable. Even these therapists must be carefully vetted and not assumed to be properly skilled. Additionally, therapists working with cops need to be skilled in the areas of psychological trauma, marriage and family, and substance misuse disorders. Sometimes those skills can be found in a single therapist, but more likely an agency will need a number of therapists to meet their needs.

Cops Like Therapists That ...

My experience observing cops' response to therapy is they are reluctant to start but become true believers and advocates afterwards. Cops respect authority, and if they believe the therapist is skilled, they are eager to follow an action plan. Cops also want to have their thinking challenged, look for feedback, insight, and direction.

What I think cops often want is to be told what to do, in other words, "If I'm the problem, I want to know. And I want something to work on." For a cop client and therapist, this could translate to an action or treatment plan. They are not interested in a therapist who passively listens until the cop figures something out. Some therapist bristles when I mention this because they claim to not tell people what to do.

Cops can be very goal oriented and have limited use for sympathy. Unlike some in society who do not feel as if they have ever been listened to, this is not the case with most cops. I have had cops complain about a therapist, saying, "All the therapist did was sit there with a sad look on his face and nod." Another told me, "She tried that active listening stuff on me." For these reasons and more, some therapists find cops to be some of the most challenging and rewarding clients to work with.

Confidentiality

Licensed therapists are legally and ethically bound to maintain a cop's privacy. The only time confidentiality can be broken is in rare situations where there is a risk of immediate serious harm to the officer or others, or cases of suspected abuse or neglect of vulnerable people such as children and the elderly. Additionally, a therapist must notify federal officials of a national security risk. Otherwise, the therapist must obtain the officer's written consent before anything that was said in counseling can be released to anyone. The only time the officer's agency has a right to know that a particular officer is attending therapy is when it is court ordered or the agency has mandated the therapy, but even in those cases, the content of the session cannot be shared.

Officers retain the right to privacy about their medications, mental health diagnosis, or even voluntary admission into a rehabilitation facility. This is not the case in mandated Fitness for Duty evaluations where the judgment and supporting information is not privileged and is accessible to the agency.

As the EAP director, I have opportunities to demonstrate confidentiality daily. For example, when people call or approach me on behalf of another and ask if I know about a particular issue or situation, answering yes or no could be a breach of confidentiality. What I have found both useful and supportive of a reputation of trustworthiness is to tell the person that we can have a one-way conversation. They tell me what they think I should know, and I internally compare it to what I do or do not know, and decide if any action is required.

Contact with EAP, or whoever arranges access to mental health resources, must remain strictly confidential, with the exception of critical incidents, which are work-related events and the involved officers are identified or known. Yet the content of any therapeutic sessions, whether it is related to a critical incident or any other issue, is not anyone else's business but the cop and the therapist. There are exceptions however when it is discovered that a client is at serious and specific risk to themselves or others. Another exception is when an officer is mandated by a supervisor to see the EAP director or a therapist, in which case the fact that the session occurred is semi-private, meaning that compliance with the direct order must be verified. However, verification is limited to a thumbs-up or thumbs-down as to whether the mandate was fulfilled.

Communications with peer support team members or the police EAP director are confidential, but not privileged. This is no different than communication with a trusted coworker or friend. Meaning, these people could be subpoenaed to testify in court. But even therapists, who are privileged, can have their records subpoenaed. As best as I can tell, most of the confidentiality concerns about officers seeking therapeutic help have not been tested in case law.

I know there is a stigma associated with seeking therapeutic help, and I respect that and continuously and vigorously treat confidentiality as my primary responsibility. But when I talk with officers at roll-calls, training sessions or other interactions, I intentionally act like there is not a stigma, meaning I do not overstate the stigma or even mention it. I do my part to lessen the stigma by instead speaking openly about common distressing issues such as depression or struggles to balance work and family life. My primary intention is to be friendly, hopeful and demonstrate a readiness to facilitate confidential access to help.

Recovery and Support

A mistake cops make is thinking in all-or-none terms, choosing to say nothing and endure further suffering in the face of a small risk. They do this even though what actually puts them at greatest risk is not getting help. When seeking professional help, the chance that something bad will happen is small, and the chance of something good is huge. Reluctance to seek help is more likely because it is hard and scary, not because something bad will happen.

Mental health problems are both common and difficult with symptoms that come and go. It can be easy to put your efforts into trying to rid yourself of your problem, whereas you should focus on managing your problem. Your task is to anticipate what thoughts and situations make things worse or better. A good goal is to feel confident and take control where you can and discover which self-care techniques and treatments work best for you.

CHAPTER 7

BEHAVIORAL HEALTH CRISIS

Officer Needs Help

IN MY 3 COLUMNS OF OFFICER DISTRESS, I defined a **behavioral health crisis** as *a loss of psychological function required to do the work.* Another description could be behavioral health chaos, a life that is dangerously out of control. This is not law enforcement specific, unique to police work, or necessarily occurred because of the work. The crisis could be related to the job, but more likely, struggles here have to do with an officer's genetics, adverse childhood experiences, ineffective coping skills, or any number of factors. In the larger field of mental health, behavioral health crisis is likely defined more broadly.

Behavioral health crises discussed in this chapter include severe depression, mental health hospitalization, suicide intention or attempt, substance use disorder detoxification or treatment facility admission. In some cases, PTSD can be a behavioral health crisis; however, I chose to describe it in more detail in the section on psychological trauma in Chapter 5. These conditions may need complex medical and psychological services. Health insurance providers can help facilitate this by assigning a behavioral health case manager to help coordinate and guide care. This can be a very useful resource to help the officer navigate services.

I wish to emphasize that all of the conditions listed as behavioral health crises are on a range of severity. Having one of these conditions does not categorically mean one cannot do the work of being a police officer, but they sure could if any of these conditions become severe enough to interfere with the job. It is best to avoid a crisis if at all possible, and remember that with expert help even these crises can be overcome.

Severe Depression or Mental Health Hospitalization

It is normal to feel sad, down or have a low mood once in a while, but feeling that way most of the time, having it persistently affect your daily life, and when it is not related to a loss or medical condition, may be an indication of severe depression. Other words used to describe severe depression are "major" or "clinical" or "debilitating." A constant sense of hopelessness and despair is a sign of severe depression. It is marked by a depressed mood most of the day, sometimes particularly in the morning, and a loss of interest in normal activities and relationships.[1] Depression becomes a behavioral health crisis when the officer is so debilitated that they are unable to work, are suicidal, or need hospitalization.

Some people can mask severe levels of depression. I have spoken to officers who have admitted there were times while working in uniform that they were so depressed they did not care whether they lived or died. This was obviously an extremely dangerous situation for all.

Hospital inpatient services support people with severe mental health problems, or people who are experiencing a crisis. Most hospital admissions are voluntary, but if you are assessed and judged to be at risk of harming yourself or others, you can be detained under an involuntary psychiatric hold. Officers should know that this is different from the Transportation Hold they may have signed as part of their police duties. The length of your hospital stay depends on how long it takes for you to stabilize or improve. Most cops probably find the thought of being hospitalized intolerable or terrifying. However, it may be their best option for expert help and safety. Some officers have said it was exactly what they needed at the time. We must act during a crisis or suspected crisis, but sometimes hospitalization can be avoided if treatment is sought earlier.

Suicide Intention or Attempt

Many people have had thoughts of suicide at some time in their lives. It is estimated that 3.7% of the U.S. population had thoughts of suicide in the past year, with 1.0% of the population developing a suicide plan and 0.5% attempting suicide.[2] When it comes to identifying a behavioral health crisis, I find it useful to differentiate between a thought of suicide, intention to suicide, or an actual attempt to die by suicide.

In patrol work, when a suicidal citizen simply admits to a thought of suicide, most commonly it results in police action on our part. Meaning, they are going to the hospital whether they like it or not. We tend to be very black and white about it, for good reason, it is beyond our ability or willingness to discern the level of risk. If, on the other hand, a police officer expresses to me thoughts of suicide, I do not want to over-react because of my own discomfort, and in effect, potentially punish him for speaking honestly about his thoughts. I do not treat the talk of suicide lightly, but neither do I let the possibility of it paralyze me. I recognize my control of another person is limited and that EAP work is not without risk. It is most important to keep the conversation going, and I do not wish to treat a thought the same as an action. This is why I was careful to describe a crisis as an intention or attempt to die by suicide.

In my job it is not uncommon to get calls from cops concerned about another cop's risk of suicide. I always follow-up, but I have also learned it can often be more about the fear of the cop who calls and her need to avoid feeling she failed to do something if the worst happens. On the other hand, I am sometimes shocked and disappointed with how bad things can get before concerned cops finally take action.

Officer Suicide Prevention

It is not clear whether police officers die by suicide more than those in other professions. We do know that more officers die by suicide than by homicide, and certain risk-taking behaviors or personal neglect may be a form of self-harm. What is clear is suicide's finality, removing all chances of recovery and burdening loved ones with the horror and loss. Of those who jumped from the Golden Gate Bridge, Kevin Hines is one of the rare survivors (less than 1%). Immediately after he leapt over the rails he recalls, "In that instant, I thought, what have I just done? I don't want to die. God, please save me."[3] and other survivors have also acknowledged instant regret.[4,5] This illustrates the importance of suicide prevention.

The exact number of officer suicides is difficult to determine, and if you consider deliberately hidden or underreported data and other factors such as the blurry line of risk-taking behavior or personal neglect, it may be unknowable. However, we can reasonably conclude this about officer suicide, it is a serious problem that appears to be increasing, and an officer is more likely to die by his own hand than the hand of another. Problems like untreated mental health issues, substance use disorders and significant relationship changes such as divorce, can put officers at greater risk.

When an officer dies by suicide, we in law enforcement feel a special pain that other professions may not, in part because we know that we did not give the same time and attention to minimize the risk of death by our own hand, as we do death at the hand of another. And we wonder if the mental and emotional armor we wear to do the job may keep us from getting help.

Feeling Helpless, Hopeless, Worthless. From the outside, depression is not always obvious and can be harder to detect as people isolate or act in hostile ways to friends and coworkers. On the inside, someone can feel helpless, hopeless, worthless and alone. On the outside, they may appear normal as some officers who died by suicide were able to hide their level of distress from coworkers. We can however form a suicide danger watch list that includes signs of depression, untreated or unmanaged alcohol problems, and relationships conflicts. In addition to this list, we should be alarmed if an officer's statements or actions, suggest he is experiencing a loss of hope, feelings of worthlessness, or feelings of not belonging or of being a burden to others.

Officer suicide prevention is complicated by myths and misconceptions about suicide as well as our own discomfort about the subject. What helped demystify it for me was learning that the primary objective might not be a wish to die, but instead relief from pain, psychic or otherwise. In some states of mind, suicide can make sense. In a presentation I attended, Dr. Robert Douglas, Jr., a former officer and the founder and executive director of the National Police Suicide Foundation, guided us through a simple exercise. He asked each of us to privately list in order of importance the three things we value the most. Someone might list marriage, family, and career. Then we were asked to imagine a circumstance where we believed all three were lost. An example could be an officer, who for whatever reason, had an extramarital affair, got caught and had to leave his home, then due to work behavior problems was fired. With this exercise, suicide suddenly felt less abstract.

I once heard about an officer, who apparently greatly valued his reputation as an honest and ethical person. He died by suicide following the decision that he was to be disciplined after it was discovered he had lied about an unintentional discharge of a Taser. There may have been more to it, but we are certainly aware that for some (teenagers for example), suicide can be a seemingly impulsive act or make sense as a result of a breakup or other seemingly transient event. We do not want to get to the point where suicide makes sense for any of our coworkers, we want them to ask us for help, and we want to know how best to respond.

It is important to be accurate about the factors that contribute to suicide. Although the study subjects were soldiers, a 2013 military report appears to reinforce the Defense Department's assertion that suicide among troops is not tied to deployment stress or combat exposure, there is no statistical connection between combat and suicide.

A comprehensive Pentagon review of military suicides has shown that more than half of the service members who died by suicide never deployed and more than 80 percent had not seen combat. The Department of Defense-backed study found that military factors — mainly deployment and combat exposure — do not appear to put troops at an increased risk for suicide. Instead, issues like mental health disorders and alcohol abuse seem to play a significant role, just as they do in civilian suicides.[6]

Therefore, we can conclude that officer suicide prevention efforts must include a focus on the larger issues of mental health, access to therapeutic resources and substance misuse treatment. Suicide prevention initiatives include talking more openly about the subject, education and dispelling myths, identifying risk factors and warning signs, recognizing and supporting protective factors, identifying resources for help, and encouraging people to act on their concerns.

Some people have thoughts of suicide that need to be expressed as they work through the related or underlying thoughts and feelings. This requires that we allow individuals to mention thoughts of suicide without fearing that just mentioning the word will result in a dramatic and decisive response. Those listening do well to differentiate between a stated thought, from an intention or an attempt to commit suicide. The later of the two require some action; the mere thought expressed should result in more conversation.

The following is a simple acronym (QPR) that can be used to guide a peer or coworker who is concerned about another's intention to die by suicide.[7]

QPR = Question persons about thoughts of suicide, **Persuade** them to seek help, **Refer** them to professional services.

The key is to ask questions about coworkers' suicidal thoughts and actions without fear that mentioning it will somehow introduce the idea to them. The act of asking questions and expressing concern may give them the hope they cannot give themselves. Intervention is connecting them with expert help.

Some officers with thoughts of suicide are at such risk that they need to be hospitalized. Experts use a line of questioning to determine if hospitalization is necessary. This questioning goes beyond the scope of concerned coworkers or peer support team members. Jack Kloss, a suicidologist, has prepared a list of questions that can give us insight into how clinicians identify suicide risk indications and the severity of risk.

> [Clinicians] may ask about the wish to die, their goal and what attracts them to the idea and what they wish to achieve. They ask about suicide planning, listening for the level of detail and access to lethal means. How the thought of suicide makes them feel paying close attention to statements about peacefulness and relief. They also inquire about protective factors, any barriers that keep them from dying by suicide. All this helps the clinician differentiate mere thoughts from intentions and assess risk. Those that show indications of impaired judgment, including substance use, are strong indications for hospitalization.[8]

The reality is that suicide can make sense to those in unbearable pain or suffering. For those who express thoughts of suicide, we engage them in a conversation about their distress and work to persuade them to get help. For those who intend to die by suicide or who have taken specific steps toward that end, we act to interrupt the destructive thoughts and get them to expert help.

Some officers are in such severe and dangerous distress, that if we get involved, at whatever level, we cannot forget our fundamental police skills, that is, know when you need uniformed police officers to intervene, including literally calling 911. We must recognize there are some situations that require breaking confidentiality and exceed our ability for discreet handling, such as when there is a risk of immediate serious harm to self or others. I understand the reason we want to keep things private, but some situations are dangerous and beyond our ability to be effective without the help of others.

When an officer dies by suicide, we all wish we had done something different. What does *doing something different* look like? I think it looks like this: talk about mental and emotional distress and how to get help, talk about drinking problems, talk about suicide.

Officer suicide prevention efforts require focusing directly on the subject. The agencies that seem to have transcended reluctance to this and have developed the most direct and comprehensive approach to officer suicide preventions are those that have suffered the greatest suicide loss and responded boldly.

An agency's goals to better respond to the risk of officer suicide include:

- Open and informed conversations about it

- Trusted, confidential and convenient access to mental health resources

- Deliberate and effective management of substance use disorders and alcohol misuse.

If we detect feelings of hopelessness, helplessness, worthlessness in ourselves we must not trust our own judgment to remain isolated, drink or to entertain ideas of suicide. Instead we must share our concern with someone. If we recognize these feelings in others, we must impose ourselves on them. All of us are capable of having an authentic talk with another cop.

Substance Use Disorder Detoxification or Treatment Facility Admission

Substance use disorder is the official diagnostic name for what we might casually refer to as alcohol and/or drug addiction or dependence. Diagnosis of this disorder need not automatically mean there is a crisis, but left untreated a crisis will most likely occur. It is a behavioral health crisis when the officer's drinking behavior has deteriorated such that medical detoxification is required to manage withdrawal. Alcohol withdrawal is a potentially life-threatening situation. Additionally, I consider treatment facility admission, whether inpatient or outpatient, a behavioral health crisis because this is such a pivotal point for an officer in his wellness trajectory.

Individuals with substance use problems must be encouraged to seek effective treatment, not hide it for fear of losing their career. Some people do lose their career, but this is more likely a result of ignoring a problem rather than seeking help for it. Often the employer does not need to know that an officer is seeking substance use treatment. Cops can go into outpatient alcohol treatment (i.e., evenings and weekends) and nobody at the department knows other than that cop and his health care facilitator. For in-patient treatment, some officers use sick time. In most cases, it is not the employer's business as long as the worker is meeting work expectations. The Family Medical Leave Act of 1993 (FMLA) is a United States labor law requiring covered employers to provide employees with job-protected and unpaid leave for qualified medical and family reasons which includes substance use disorders. Chapter 8 goes into detail about alcohol misuse.

Fitness for Duty

Certain conditions and events may require mandated Fitness for Duty assessment, which refers to a formal process to determine if an officer is mentally and physically fit to maintain their police powers. A licensed psychologist/psychiatrist conducts the Fitness for Duty assessment. This assessment is very different from the therapeutic process and the two do not mix as discussed in Chapter 6. The Fitness for Duty process takes several hours of assessment and psychological forensics work to complete and results in a report and recommendation for the chief.

Understandably, for cops, Fitness for Duty is synonymous with not being able to be a cop, and we can be very guarded if not hostile about the topic. I have a softer way of describing it as, "They want their stuff back until you get better." The stuff is the stuff that gives you police powers and access to the police building (at our agency, it would be department issued pistol, badge and ID card). As a sign of good faith, our police department keeps the officer's badge and does not give it to anyone else until they either return or are separated. Of note, loss of your police powers could mean loss of the ability to carry a firearm if your police ID is your only 'permit to carry.' On a very rare occasion, and with the officer's complete knowledge, and sometimes encouragement, I have needed to contact their supervisor about the officer's serious risk to herself or others, or request that an officer be relieved of her work duty.

Further, it should be stated that cops should remain fit for duty and this expectation is generally reasonable and necessary. Not everyone who is a cop should be a cop, and some have neglected their health and wellbeing to such a degree that they are at risk to themselves and others. Others have, as a colleague has described, "broken about four or five of the Ten Commandments, and now demand endless resources and to be absolved of all their wrongdoings." It should not work that way, and it is unfair to the earnest cops.

Note: State law enforcement licensing or oversight boards/agencies generally set standards regarding eligibility, hiring, and training, as well as enforce license eligibility following criminal convictions. Mental health and fitness for duty issues are the purview of individual police agencies.

Disappearing Cops

Less dramatic, and not necessarily a behavioral health crisis, but still impactful, is what I call separation grief and loss, when a cop appears to suddenly disappear from the ranks due to debilitating injury, illness, discipline, getting fired or in some cases retirement. For that cop, there can be the additional distress of no longer being a cop, for those left behind, it is what appears like a sudden and unceremonious disappearance, often with bitterness about how they were treated. It might be described euphemistically as a bad death, in large part because of a lack of separation rituals.

Once an officer asked me to clean out his locker, he was too ashamed to be seen at work upon his eventual medical retirement. Furthermore, he had isolated himself in all ways from coworkers during his mental and emotional decline. I met him in a parking lot on the edge of the city to hand over a big plastic garbage bag of his stuff. The lack of ceremony or ritual felt grotesque and painfully inadequate for someone who had taken so much pride in being a police officer. *(Story retold with officer's permission.)*

Police work can be hard on the body and mind, some suffer serious harm due to no great fault of their own, some due to negligence and neglect. Disregarding the culpability, police work is filled with those who decline and eventually become unfit for duty or get caught up in some controversy and get fired or criminally charged. The hardship of this is great. As an EAP director or peer support team member, it is our duty to remove any judgment and reach out to them. It is important to recognize these struggles and separations are extremely lonely. Part of the reason we might avoid troubled officers is that they can become unpleasant and disagreeable people like anyone suffering. Also, we may fear these officers, as if we ourselves are one call or event away from becoming them ourselves.

We may not be able to fix a troubled officer or return them to their former selves, but we can ease their suffering by acknowledging the hardship, offering hope, aid in recovery, and in some cases honor them with a respectful separation.

Crisis Planning

We are in the crisis business, yet we may fail to prepare for the crises within our own agencies, and sometimes we have only one chance to get it right and God help the chief, supervisor or coworker who gets it wrong. An agency must consider beforehand how to respond to cops with drinking problems, suicide intentions, severe depression or need for mental health hospitalization, as well as meeting the mental health needs of an officer arrested for DWI or domestic violence for example.

A supervisor cannot be expected to be proficient at all things and must carefully consider when and when not to act, but when it concerns behavioral health crises, such as debilitating or unmanaged depression and officer suicide prevention, the supervisor must act. A good supervisor anticipates and plans for things, and certain behavioral health crises must be included in that planning. This includes knowing what expert help to seek, and how exactly to reach them when needed.

Response to these issues commonly involves utilization of an officer's health insurance plan. Concerns about how accessing insurance impacts future employment should not be dismissed; however, officers need to be reminded that getting help does not cost them their jobs, but failing to get help definitely can.

The supervisor's role is to be accessible and reassuring, and to connect people with the help they need. A responsible and potentially lifesaving response includes recognizing some situations go beyond our abilities, and officers may be in immediate danger.

Many crises are predictable and thus often preventable. Yet, as much as we would like to get ahead of the crisis, we must know that our job as helpers and friends is to maintain trustworthiness and be responsive and effective when a crisis does occur. This requires planning and continuous messages of both warning and successful recovery. As we work toward harm reduction and prevention, we should know that the impact might not be realized until the crisis nears or arrives, and hopefully then those in crisis will reach out and we will be well prepared.

CHAPTER 8

ALCOHOL

We Drink to Feel Different

I ONCE READ A NEWSPAPER STORY where a woman described seeing some famous rock star washing his clothes at a laundromat on west Seventh Street not far from downtown Saint Paul. She happened to know he was in town performing. The conclusion was that doing his own laundry was part of his sobriety, living soulfully, caring for himself by doing what ordinary people do. He, like many who lived years dependent on drugs or alcohol, lost a lot. But in recovery, people gain as well.

I recognize that successfully recovering "addicts" must know something the rest of us do not. When I am amongst a group of alcoholics in recovery, they have a look in their eyes when they greet each other, a kind of knowing, a bond. Some members of this group appear more grateful, but still wary of the spark and fire that consumes. They have suffered, often publicly, forced to go deeply into themselves where they discovered that there was more. I come at this topic from a helper point of view, not as someone who is in recovery. I say this because I recognize that people in recovery tell their own story best. Some of the people I admire most in life are people who are in recovery from alcohol or other drug addictions, who have gone through a kind of hell and survived.

This chapter will focus on alcohol problems and is influenced by *Facing Addiction in America: The Surgeon General's Report on Alcohol, Drugs and Health*, 2016. You will learn that what we commonly think of as drinking problems or alcoholism is now described as a substance use disorder, a chronic illness which can be prevented and treated with expert help and peer support. Yet, in its most severe cases, addiction, left untreated likely results in death, and a lot of wreckage on the way down. An airline pilot in recovery gave thanks by saying, "Successful recovery for some means they get to live a life they almost threw away: get to wear the uniform again, remain married, maintain their kids love and respect, and you did not die like my parents did."[1] Dealing effectively with a cop's alcohol problem requires not only an understanding of the science of addiction and treatment, but insight into the heart and mind of the police officer and workplace.

Feel Different

Once while driving I reached down to turn on the radio, only to discover that it was already on. I had done this a few times before. Curious, this time I paused and backtracked to see what I had been thinking and feeling. I realized I was anxious and was looking to be distracted from my own thoughts. This is a mild example, but we do this in ways big and small: when we feel bored, disappointed, depressed, sad, or bad in some way, we seek something that will make us feel different. The list of things that can do this for us are varied and personal, healthy and unhealthy. If a cop's goal is to unwind, fall asleep more easily, or gain acceptance by the group, alcohol is a ready accomplice. From a practical point of view, alcohol is very effective in meeting these short-term goals, so much so that for some, drinking can feel like an essential element of survival. If cops did not find drinking useful to meet some essential need, then they would not be doing it. *Choir practice* may have changed over the years but using alcohol to be accepted by the group and feel different has not. Over time, drinking trains the brain and the need to feel different can become the need to feel less sick, less anxious, less bad.

My Point of View

I grew up with a deep distrust of any external means to feel different. This may have come from being the second generation of an adult child of an alcoholic, I had internalized my mother's stories of, as a little girl, retrieving her father from the bar and trying to right her household by finding his hidden liquor and pouring it down the sink.

I know lots of cops who are in sobriety, but I am gravely concerned that this group is too small. Too many cops are problem drinkers, going untreated and slowly getting worse. It is clear that we need a more systematic and science-based approach to the alcohol problem among police officers, from education, to intervention, to treatment and after-care. It was obvious to me as the EAP director that I needed to partner with internal and external experts to educate myself and to illuminate the issue within the department, so we could be more practical, straightforward, and intentional about substance use disorders.

Alcohol Focus

Alcohol is a simple drug that we can have a complicated relationship with. It is legal, readily available, socially acceptable and well ingrained in the police culture.

Certainly, there are cops who are addicted to illicit drugs and misuse prescription medications. Opioid addiction among cops likely has its origins in pain management as it does with much of society. And we could just as well be talking about other addictions, such as gambling, but because my intention is to focus more on the *why* and *how* rather than the *what*, alcohol misuse will be the subject, which I believe is the most common substance of both relief and trouble.

Alcohol use disorders do not occur immediately but over time, with repeated misuse and often gradual development of symptoms. Police officers, being law-abiding adults with careers, are generally not at risk for the immediate and direct consequences of new exposure and experimentation with alcohol or other drugs. They are more affected by alcohol's long-term physical and mental health effects and societal consequences.

Alcohol problems rightly get our attention because its destructive power is great. I have encountered plenty of cops who have impressed me on how suspicious they are about alcohol use, refraining when they suspect it would not be good for them. Some key insights from the Grant Study found that alcoholism was the main cause of divorce and strongly correlates with neurosis and depression, which tended to follow alcohol abuse, rather than precede it. Together with associated cigarette smoking, alcoholism was the single greatest contributor to early morbidity and death.[2]

Science Focus

With my health education degree and years of witnessing the ravages of alcohol as a paramedic and police officer, I thought I had a good understanding of the disease. What I discovered was that my understanding was superficial. Interestingly, those suffering addiction obviously know the experience of it, but even they often lack even a basic understanding of the brain science and the addiction cycle that drives it. In this chapter, I will describe the addiction cycle, much of which might be applicable to some of the other "vices" people use to feel different, including: tobacco, gambling, food, sex, pornography, internet/social media, video games, working, shopping, and others.

Including information on the science of addiction helps us reframe the subject of alcohol misuse and abuse by focusing our attention on the brain and away from questions of morality, moral failing, or character weakness and flaws. Failure and weakness are fighting words to cops. With a scientific perspective, we develop curiosity about the chemical attributes of a particular substance and how the brain works. We can also gain some sympathy towards those who are born with an increased susceptibility to the problem. Knowing that alcohol and other drugs can change the brain's circuitry, we see how sobriety is more than a matter of willpower. Substance use disorder is a chronic illness that is preventable and treatable. An accurate understanding of the brain's reward system, and a compassionate and systematic application of the science of addiction will lessen the stigma and shame, so we can be more practical and purposeful in how we approach the problem.

"All things be ready if your mind be so" is a quote credited to both Shakespeare and Dizzy Gillespie. Equally important to understanding the science of addiction and treatment is to get your mind right about the officer, the workplace, help, and the role of helper. Agencies must focus on education and early intervention in addition to responding to those who ask for and need help.

How Much Is Too Much? Assessing Your Drinking Behavior

Alcohol problems can progress slowly and in many cases the cop will not be the best judge of the severity of the problem or the negative impact of his drinking. This chapter includes a detailed description of the science of addiction and treatment. However, the central question for many is, "Am I drinking too much?" or "Do I have a drinking problem?" What follows is an example of assessment questions from the National Institute on Alcohol Abuse and Alcoholism that can help you explore this concern. For an online assessment with immediate feedback go to www .rethinkingdrinking.niaaa.nih.gov.[3]

In the past year, have you:

- Had times when you ended up drinking more, or longer, than you intended?

- More than once wanted to cut down or stop drinking, or tried to, but couldn't?

- More than once gotten into situations while or after drinking that increased your chances of getting hurt (such as driving, swimming, using machinery, walking in a dangerous area, or having unsafe sex)?

- Had to drink much more than you once did to get the effect you want? Or found that your usual number of drinks had much less effect than before?

- Continued to drink even though it was making you feel depressed or anxious or adding to another health problem? Or after having had a memory blackout?

- Spent a lot of time drinking? Or being sick or getting over other aftereffects?

- Continued to drink even though it was causing trouble with your family or friends?

- Found that drinking — or being sick from drinking — often interfered with taking care of your home or family? Or caused job troubles? Or school problems?

- Given up or cut back on activities that were important or interesting to you, or gave you pleasure, in order to drink?

- More than once gotten arrested, been held at a police station, or had other legal problems because of your drinking?

- Found that when the effects of alcohol were wearing off, you had withdrawal symptoms, such as trouble sleeping, shakiness, restlessness, nausea, sweating, a racing heart, or a seizure? Or sensed things that were not there?

Source: National Institute on Alcohol Abuse and Alcoholism, Rethinking Drinking.

One measurement for problem drinking behavior is binge drinking which is defined as, "for men, drinking 5 or more standard alcoholic drinks, and for women, 4 or more on the same occasion on at least 1 day in the past 30 days."[4] Beyond the definition of binge drinking, there is evidence to support that there is "no significant difference between men and women in the amount of alcohol that can be consumed without a drop in life expectancy." The science on alcohol limits seems to be shifting, but currently, the threshold for low-risk drinking is seven beers a week for both men and women.[5] No-risk drinking is zero beers a week.

Police Culture

Gravity Attack

When doing public safety work, it can seem like everyone is drunk or high. We get called when people under the influence fall down, crash into things, punch, bite or shoot each other. When I was working as a paramedic, there were days in which it seemed every patient's illness or injury was related to alcohol use, both chronic and acute. As an urban ambulance worker, calls for "one-down" were ten times more likely to be a wino than some heart attack victim; I use to refer to them as gravity attacks. We even took trips from the ER hauling a half-dozen drunks at a time to detox when the ER needed more beds. It was so common to be charting something about alcohol that we used its shorthand, "ETOH" (EtOH is chemical abbreviation for ethyl/ethanol) which in a career's time might save an hour or two of writing.

As a cop, it was the same or worse. There were calls when the suspect was drunk, the victim was drunk, the witnesses were drunk, and this is the part of the story where I am supposed to say that one of the cops was drunk, but I won't. In fact, I used to get a laugh out of a crowd with the argument, "Listen, I'm the only one sober here, let me make the decisions."

As society suffers, so do the police. Life can be difficult — at times extremely difficult. We drink to feel different, and drinking can have very practical applications, though like any shortcut, it has its own hazards and negative consequences.

Plenty of cops drink too much, but it is unclear if police officers abuse alcohol more than others. "Despite the widely held assumption that police officers are at risk for higher-than-average rates of alcohol abuse, very little research has been conducted to investigate patterns of substance abuse within the law enforcement field."[6] No matter the rate, the consequences for cops' misuse may be more severe and treatment more challenging because of the closed nature of the group, occupational necessity to distrust others, and risks associated with revealing any vulnerability. It does appear that cops binge drink more than others, and many cops use alcohol to unwind and to fall asleep.[7]

The Cops

Patrol cops judge each other's competence for both personal and group survival. They need assurances that another cop is a committed member of the group. They rightly fear anything lacking may signal to their coworkers that they are a liability or cannot be trusted. Simultaneously, they know that exposing a weakness on the street creates a vulnerability that will be seized upon by those who would do them harm.

The cop is a suspicious creature, for good reason. Building trust with police officers includes not trying to talk them out of stuff they think or know they need. Approaching strangers for a living requires that they be stingy with trust and advantage themselves against sudden violence by taking control whenever possible. And cops get good at it. Being necessarily strong and tough, cautious and suspicious of those outside the group can be supremely useful in police work, but can get over developed, misapplied, and can have serious negative consequences in our personal lives and hinder our willingness to seek good help. It is most useful to help cops see that some of the things causing them trouble are often normal adaptations, necessary adjustments made for mental, emotional, and physical survival. But we can also remind them that they have learned some things that can both help and hurt them. For cops, their alarms have been muted, and the natural human impulse to ask for help may have been suppressed. All of this may be summarized to explain why our police culture creates barriers for officers seeking help and treatment for substance use disorders.

The Workplace

In the workplace, it is often obvious to the cops which officers are problem drinkers or full-blown alcoholics. When the troubled cop shows up late or calls in sick, other officers know why. Some troubled cops may be loners, hiding their disease by avoiding contact with coworkers and supervisors. When the supervisors fail to respond to what seem like obvious signs of trouble, cops are left asking themselves *"How are they getting away with this? Doesn't anyone notice what a mess she is?" "Is the boss being played for a fool or is he just avoiding a hard thing?"*

Others may support inaction because of a sense of loyalty and wishing to protect the cop. While acknowledging that people have rights, including the right to self-harm, not acting is also acting and has its own cause-and-effect. Whether the police department's response is effective through deliberate action, or ineffective because of neglect of duty, supervisors must know all officers are closely watching. Sometimes what is most glaring is that the obvious is ignored.

With appropriate effort and planning, any agency can design an effective response to alcohol problems by starting where they are, using what they have, and doing what they can. That includes partnering with sober cops, learning about the science of addiction, and consulting treatment experts. At the same time, they can help those treatment centers gain a better understanding of the personality and character traits common to police officers and the police culture.

High-functioning Workplace

Getting your mind right about the workplace has more to do with the work than with the worker. The police department is primarily a workplace where we have both an individual and shared purpose and function. This includes both running towards danger and numerous mundane tasks. If a cop does not figure out that the work is not just about *their* needs, but also the needs of the community, the police force, and the labor that needs to be done, then they become part of the problem.

When considering how to manage alcohol problems among our fellow officers, know that probably the single best thing an agency can do to support the mental health and wellbeing of police officers is to have a high-functioning police department. This is a place that mostly functions well and makes sense, where decreasing uncertainty and increasing predictability reduces stress. Officers need stable ground on which to stand, especially during times of great flux, with a *few* clear expectations that are well communicated and consistently attended to. Boundaries and clear expectations are good; people, especially those in distress, need to be able to reach out and touch something solid, immovable. A high-functioning workplace is extremely important, independent of how we deal or do not deal with addiction.

It seems reasonable to expect that the chief and his command staff's primary mission is to keep the place shipshape, in good order, trim and neat. A healthy environment is most important. A study of centenarians (people living past 100) found the most beneficial thing was living in a healthy environment, where your neighbors and friends practice healthy behavior.[8] Raising the expectation of wellbeing has a positive contagious effect.

The reality is, some workplaces are disaster areas, a ship that lists badly. Though I avoid the phrase, many describe the police department as a family. I reluctantly accept the analogy only if the description includes dysfunctional families, like most. In these cases, and for their own sanity, individuals might seek out a healthy microenvironment or at least know what they are competing against. Some of the strongest support groups or networks exist within, or because of, dysfunctional environments.

The workplace is like a living organism whose health and wellbeing needs constant attention. Seemingly little things can have big meaning and failing to recognize this concept can add to a sense of disorder and lack of discipline. In the workplace, the focus needs to be on the work that needs to be done and this becomes crucial when dealing with officers with substance use disorders.

Science of Addiction and Treatment

The Problem

In 1964, the Surgeon General issued the first Report on Smoking and Health. At the time, people smoked in restaurants, movie theaters and Greyhound buses. I was a small boy then, and my father was a smoker. My father, God bless him, was completely dedicated to his family and the wellbeing of his children. He also brought home candy cigarettes for us. Soon after the report came out, he quit smoking, but said that he craved a good cigar the rest of his life. What is amazing is how common smoking was and how successfully our society changed this behavior. In 2016, the Surgeon General released the first-ever report on addiction — *Facing Addiction in America – The Surgeon General's Report on Alcohol, Drugs, and Health.*

I did not once see the word "alcoholism," "alcoholic," or "drug addict" in the massive Surgeon General's report. These terms have become antiquated, pejorative and tend to lead to all-or-none, black-and-white thinking about the problem. Instead the term substance use disorders is used, and more specifically, *alcohol use disorder.*

Most people who misuse substances do not develop a substance use disorder; however, about one in seven do.[9,10,11] This depends on a number of factors, such as a person's genetic makeup (between 40–70 percent), the age when use began, their personality and life history. Environmental and social factors, including the household dynamics and police cultures, also play a role. Some of these same factors can be protective and provide a sort of buffer against addiction and aid with recovery.[12]

The Surgeon General's report states substance use disorders occur when a person uses alcohol or drugs to such an extent that it causes clinically significant impairments in health, social functioning, and voluntary control over substance use.[13] In other words, demonstrative negative consequences such as being unable to fulfill family or work obligations, experiencing legal trouble, or engaging in hazardous behavior as a result of drug use.[14] So, if your first thought when you wake up is to wonder whom you may have offended or hurt, you probably have a problem. Of all the people with "substance use disorders only about 10 percent receive any special kind of treatment,"[15] Unfortunately this suggests only a small fraction of those in need of help seek or receive it.

Despite great progress altering our health trajectory due to all kinds of medical advances, life expectancy in the United States has plateaued or decreased for some segments of the population, due in large part to substance misuse and physical and mental health problems.[16] Alcohol misuse and alcohol use disorders alone costs the United States approximately $249 billion in lost productivity, health care expenses, law enforcement, and other criminal justice costs.[17] That comes to "about $2.05 per drink."[18]

Cops are already busy helping society, we do that for a living, we need to learn about substance misuse and the science of addiction so we can help ourselves and other cops. The science of addiction and treatment is fascinating, and despite having plenty of direct experience dealing with drunks and the results of intoxication, you may be surprised by how little you really understand about the disease. With this knowledge, you will know what you are up against.

The Brain and Substance Use

Feel Good and Repeat

We interact with the world and the world interacts with us. Seeking pleasure and avoiding displeasure keeps both the individual and species alive. The reward of a pleasure experience is a chemical process in the brain that motivates people to continue to engage in these activities. Likewise, pain or displeasure motivates us to avoid things. This system can become hijacked by anything associated with pleasure or pain and can lead to the addiction cycle. Four behaviors are central to the addiction cycle: [19]

- impulsivity,

- positive reinforcement,

- negative reinforcement,

- compulsivity.

Impulsivity is when we partake in something with little or no regard to future consequences. We will seek it and repeat it if the experience gives us pleasure (**positive reinforcement**) or if it helps us avoid displeasure (**negative reinforcement**), even if temporary or short-lived.[20]

Impulsivity shifts to **compulsivity**, as the user is increasingly driven less by positive reinforcement (feeling pleasure) and more by negative reinforcement (feeling relief). Negative reinforcement occurs when a person drinks to relieve discomfort of the buzz wearing off or to get rid of the withdrawal symptoms in the absence of alcohol (or any other substance). These withdrawal symptoms can include stress, anxiety, depression, or physical illness. "Eventually, the person begins taking the substance not to get "high," but rather to escape the "low" feelings to which, ironically, chronic drug use has contributed. Compulsive substance seeking is a key characteristic of addiction, as is the loss of control over use. Compulsivity helps to explain why many people with addiction experience relapses after attempting to abstain from or reduce use."[21]

With repeated use, the positive reinforcing effects fade and the user may develop a tolerance that requires increasing amounts of the substance to get the same affect. As police officers, we can certainly recall the thrill and excitement of events and activities that are now more routine or at least much less exciting. Some officers openly admit that they are, or were, adrenalin junkies. But over time it takes more and more to get them excited. This is also known as chasing the high, a potentially unobtainable goal — as the saying goes, there is nothing more dissatisfying than almost enough. For the addict, they need the substance to feel better or less bad. Overcoming tolerance and fending off withdrawal symptoms becomes a full-time occupation demanding more and more attention. Additional attention is devoted to hiding the addiction or making excuses for all the other things in their lives that are neglected, as they are subservient to their first love, alcohol.

The Brain

The brain is constantly sorting out what has meaning and what does not, and this activity is mostly subconscious and automatic. Continuously, connections between certain brain cells are being strengthened or allowed to fade away. The sum of all this activity constitutes how the brain works. The brain is composed of nerve cells (neurons) which are organized in groups of neuronal networks that perform all kinds of specific functions. The neurons communicate with each other through chemical messengers called neurotransmitters. Addiction can be thought of as a brain disease or disorder because the addiction cycle disrupts the normal functions of some of these neuronal networks.[22]

In the discussion in Chapter 5 regarding psychological trauma, I describe the brain as if it has two parts, the animal brain and the human brain. To better understand the development and persistence of substance use disorders, it is useful to focus on three regions of the brain. The basal ganglia and the amygdala are within the animal or non-thinking brain, and the prefrontal cortex is part of the human or thinking brain.

The animal brain parts (basal ganglia and extended amygdala) are involved in such things as:

- Coordination

- Routines and habits

- Motivation and reward

- Regulating reactions to stress or negative emotions.

The human brain parts (prefrontal cortex) are involved in higher functions such as:

- Organizing thoughts and activities, prioritizing tasks and managing time

- Decision making

- Regulating actions, emotions, and impulses.[23,24]

All addictive substances have powerful effects on the entire brain. As a person continues to misuse alcohol or other substances, progressive changes, or adaptations, occur in the structure and function of the brain. These changes alter how a person processes pleasure, learns, manages stress, makes decisions, and maintains self-control. The brain changes continue long after the person stops using substances producing what we commonly think of as cravings.[25]

The Addiction Cycle

Addiction can be described as a three-stage cycle that repeats itself over and over again. Although addiction can include gambling, shopping, sex or any number of activities or substances, I will use alcohol in the description of the addiction cycle.

1. Binge/intoxication – feels good or feels less bad

2. Withdrawal/negative affect – want or need more

3. Preoccupation/anticipation – it is all I can think about.[26]

Stage 1. Binge/Intoxication

In this stage, the person consumes an intoxicating substance and experiences its rewarding or pleasurable effects. The animal brain responds by producing a pleasure surge of the neurotransmitter dopamine. This is very pleasurable and the brain links the alcohol, or anything associated, with the reward. Certain moods, people or places, even the sound of a clinking glass can trigger substance seeking as the user has retrained the brain.[27]

Stage 2. Withdrawal/Negative Affect

In the absence of alcohol, a person experiences negative emotions and, sometimes, symptoms of physical illness. The negative feelings associated with withdrawal are thought to come from diminished activation in the reward circuitry and activation of the brain's stress systems.[28]

As substance use increases, the brain attempts to maintain balance by adapting and establishing a "new normal." The brain circuits scale back their sensitivity to dopamine, leading to a reduction in alcohol's ability to produce euphoria or the "high" that comes from using it. Because these same circuits are involved in our ability to take pleasure from ordinary rewards like food, sex, and social interaction, the consequence can be that the rest of life can feel less and less enjoyable.[29,30] Good feelings feel less good and are increasingly harder to reach, while at the same time the bad feelings increase in frequency and intensity. This explains why those in recovery often describe a renewed enjoyment of simple pleasures and a return to a life with more choices, one that is not dominated by being lured towards pleasure and pushed to escape pain.[31]

In patrol work, we see dramatic examples of this in the people we deal with, especially as the intensity of their drug of choice increases, such as seen with the arrival of crack and meth. An old cop told me that they used to spend their time patrolling alleys hoping to catch burglars, which seems antiquated now with high call volumes and bold violent criminal behavior. The nature and intensity of policing changed with the nature and intensity of drug use.

Stage 3. Preoccupation/Anticipation

The first two stages involve the animal brain, automatic things, or subconscious reactions. The third stage involves the human brain, how we think, make decisions, achieve goals and manage desires and wants.[32] In this stage the person becomes preoccupied with alcohol, either drinking or thinking about drinking. Healthy people can balance these "animal brain" impulses with judgment and reason that reside in the prefrontal cortex. Unfortunately, for those with substance use disorders, the circuits of the big thinking brain that could otherwise make better decisions are disrupted. The result is poor or compromised self-control.[33]

Cops should be rightly concerned about their drinking if they started drinking very young, have a genetic predisposition (meaning a close relative has a substance use disorder), or have had negative consequences from their drinking. Understanding the brain science and the cycle of addiction helps us see that alcohol use disorder is a chronic and progressive brain disease that will not get better on its own, and takes more than willpower to overcome, and requires expert help.

Co-occurring Disorders

Co-occurring means two or more problems existing at the same time. It is important to recognize this because successful recovery may depend on treatment of both problems or illnesses. It is not uncommon for a person with a substance use disorder to also have other disorders such as anxiety or depression. The reasons for this overlap could be due to a number of factors and having one mental disorder could increase vulnerability for another. A substance use disorder could trigger a mental disorder that would otherwise not have occurred.[34] For example, "research suggests that alcohol use increases risk for PTSD by altering the brain's ability to recover from traumatic experiences." [35,36] Conversely, having a mental health disorder may cause a person to "self-medicate" using alcohol, as a way of attempting to cope with the symptoms of the disorder. It is also possible that substance use disorders and mental disorders are "caused by shared, overlapping factors, such as particular genes, neurobiological deficits, and exposure to traumatic or stressful life experiences."[37] Therefore, successful treatment starts with an accurate assessment of the problem or often interrelated problems.

Assessment and Treatment

Assessment and Diagnosis

Alcohol misuse, or full-blown dependence and addiction, like most other medical illness, can range from mild to severe. The progression from mild, moderate to severe is predictable and yet can be deceptively gradual. What makes things problematic is the user can be the worst judge of his own behavior for a number of reasons, such as the perceived need to rationalize behavior and that chronic alcohol use, as demonstrated by the addiction cycle, can hijack the brain and impair thinking and decision making.[38] An honest and accurate assessment likely requires a neutral trained profession, but a useful self-assessment can begin in the privacy of one's own home using simple on-line resources. This can be followed-up with a professional assessment, and if needed, a treatment plan recommendation. Ultimately, trained professionals who conduct a clinical interview using standardized questions make the diagnosis of a substance use disorder. The result is a treatment plan that generally requires only small changes for mild problems, moderate changes for moderate problems, and severe or intense treatment for severe problems.[39]

Many people may think of treatment as simply stopping drinking. Although that is obviously part of the process, recovery involves many stages. The stopping drinking part can be medically hazardous and needs to be managed, especially for those with heavy alcohol use. Detoxification, or maybe a better term, acute stabilization, is needed to manage the physical and emotional symptoms that occur after a person stops drinking. Stabilization may be thought of as first in a series of steps towards recovery.[40]

Treatment

There are different treatment and recovery programs that emphasis different things, such as Alcoholics Anonymous (AA) or Self-Management and Recovery Training (SMART) as well as others. AA or Twelve-Step programs are not a form of treatment, but instead a means of on-going recovery support.[41] Members share a common problem or status, learn from each other, and focus on personal change goals.[42] Recovery groups can provide a "new social setting in which former alcohol or drug users can engage with others in the absence of substance related cues from their former life."[43] A "place" to practice accountability and the necessary skills to living sober. The groups are voluntary associations that charge no fees and are self-led by the members. For many, there is a spiritual element and one that includes the help of anonymous "strangers."

For many, SMART Recovery represents an alternative to AA. SMART is a support program that is solely science or evidence-based, secular and utilizes cognitive behavioral therapy (CBT) which focuses on developing coping strategies by deepening an understanding of the connection between behavior, thoughts and feelings. Some have described AA and Twelve-Step programs as outward looking, and SMART or similar programs as inward looking.

The severity and complexity of a person's drinking problem will dictate the recommended treatment plan. In all cases, the goals are similar to treating any medical condition: return them to full-functioning by reducing major symptoms and strengthen them against a return to the problem. Based on the input of professionals, fellow people in sobriety, or through their own self-discovery, some people realize that this means completely abstaining from alcohol.[44]

It can take a year of abstinence from alcohol before a person can be said to be in remission (recovery). It may take 4 to 5 years of abstinence before a person's risk of relapse lessens to match the general population's risk of developing a substance use disorder during their lifetime.[45]

While intensive treatment may be required for some cops, often less intense counseling and outpatient management is more appropriate. The term "functional alcoholic" is a misnomer in that an alcohol use disorder is a progressive disease and just because someone is able to show up at work and not get fired, does not mean they are functioning well, or at all, in all areas of their lives.

Cop-Only verses Mixed-Group Treatment. I have heard differing opinions and experiences regarding cop-only treatment and support groups. It seems very reasonable that a cop could be very concerned about commingling with non-cops and potential "criminals" while seeking treatment and recovery. This is a perception about safety during a time of increased vulnerability. Being in close quarters, mentally and physically, with those who you may not trust, or who may recognize you as a cop, or you would arrest if circumstances were different, will no doubt make things difficult.

Even if cop-only groups were desired, in most regions it cannot be reliably accommodated. Police are estranged in society, yet we are more alike than we are different. Part of the path to recovery is seeing what you have in common with others who are similarly addicted. There is a profound benefit to being humbled by your addiction and the experience of being accepted by non-cops could be part of the joy of sobriety.

Behavioral and Family Therapy

For some, it took years to develop a substance use disorder and much of their thinking, routines, and social interactions are linked to their drinking. In other words, they have lived a significant portion of their lives with drinking as a central part. Thus, it should not surprise people that it can take multiple layers of support, daily attention to sobriety and years of abstinence to reach a state of relative stability. But over time, a moment-to-moment struggle and daily practice of new behaviors, can give way to weekly maintenance practices and then an extended period of time of enjoying living sober. For some, "remission is the end of a chapter in their life that they rarely think about later, if at all. But for others, particularly those with more severe substance use disorders, remission is a component of a broader change in their behavior, outlook, and identity. That change process becomes an ongoing part of how they think about themselves."[46]

Part of that journey is seeing more clearly the impact of their behavior both on their lives and the lives of their loved ones. Recovery is about more than just not drinking, and requires an examination of old behaviors, underlying issues and learning new behaviors. This can include a well-established therapeutic process described as behavioral therapy, in which participants improve coping strategies and healthy life skills.

Family members of police officers endure sacrifices that are not required of most other professions. The addition of a household member with a substance use disorder only adds additional stress. Addiction is a family illness, and recovery must involve the entire family who will need to rebuild a life that may have been damaged by years of neglect and abuse. The positive changes that occur when a household member achieves sobriety can significantly change the previously established roles and expectations. The newly sober member, the parent for example, might in effect become a fully functioning member again. Changes, even the positive changes related to sobriety, will lead to other changes, and disrupt the balance and dynamics of the entire household. Spouses of returning soldiers may experience this when the previously absent parent returns and takes on parental duties that were previously managed without them. For a household, maybe previously dominated by actions and consequences of a substance use disorder, all members will need help with adjustment.

Al-Anon

I probably refer as many or more people to Al-Anon as I do problem drinkers to assessment for possible treatment. Al-Anon is a mutual support program for people whose lives are affected by someone else's drinking. I am more likely to get a call from a problem drinker's close friend, partner or loved one than I am from the problem drinker. I tell these people that I am very willing to reach out to the person they are concerned about, but if the problem drinker is not the one calling me, I tell them I recognize the limited power I have to influence change. I then switch the conversation to them. Possibly the best support for a person in distress is to support the supporter and I encourage them to seek the help *they* need. Groups such as Al-Anon can help a friend or loved one "systematically and strategically alter their own unproductive behaviors that have emerged in their efforts to deal with the substance use problems of their affected loved one."[47] The primary goal is to help participants build internal strength and stability. Support them in building the skills needed for "loving detachment" from the loved one rather than focusing on how to get their loved one into treatment.[48]

Recovery and Wellness

Although recovery is a very personal journey, those in recovery have discovered interdependence, and recognize a debt they owe to others or those who have gone before them. Just the knowing that recovery is attainable and being modeled for them by those who have been successful is helpful.

Both the individual officer and the agency do well to view substance use disorders as both a serious medical condition and one that can be very successfully treated. Agencies contribute to recovery by acknowledging the problem. Through thoughtful, systematic and deliberate action the agency can maintain a positive and hopeful attitude in education, assessment, treatment and aftercare.

Relapse is not uncommon or completely unexpected for some. Though potentially hazardous and disappointing, it does not mean all progress is lost. As a patrolman, there were people I took to jail for whatever reason who were so discouraged and self-loathing that I felt the need to give them a pep talk. Yes, they needed to be accountable for what they did or did not do, but all life progress was not lost, it was simply a set-back. Once recovery starts, the earnest person is never the same. Even a little self-awareness and personal insight means you are a different person, you never go all the way back to who you were before.

Ultimately, for many, recovery is a tremendous growth experience where they identify abstinence, personal growth and service to others as primary components of their success.[49] Cops in recovery may have initially feared living sober but discovered all the other elements of their life they had been missing out on because they were drunk or thinking about drinking. They may have feared returning to work after treatment, but found they were welcomed back and now a better employee than when they left for treatment. Recovered cops may enjoy most being in charge of their own life again.

Changing the Culture

One of the recurring themes in the 2016 Surgeon General's Report is that sound scientific knowledge about how to address substance use disorders effectively has outpaced society's ability and, in some cases, willingness to implement that knowledge. Agencies can implement practices that would identify and treat, but also prevent alcohol misuse from escalating to addiction. Making this change will require a cultural shift in the way officers think about, talk about, look at, and act toward people with substance use disorders. Negative public attitudes about substance misuse and use disorders can be entrenched, but it is possible to change social viewpoints. This has been done many times in the past: cancer used to be surrounded by fear and judgment, now it is regarded by many as simply a medical condition. This has helped people become comfortable talking about their concerns with their doctors, widening access to prevention and treatment.[50]

Early Intervention

Our response to drinking problems in law enforcement has largely been focused on getting the problem drinker into treatment, the 28-day "spin-dry." No pre-event education or aftercare, just wait until they crash and burn, and send them to treatment with a pat on the back while saying, "Good luck buddy." The classic inpatient treatment is more about stabilization. Experts in the field outline a detailed, systematic, and lengthy approach. Other industries, such as the airline industry for example, take an assertive and science-based approach, in effect saying, "We want you here, you are valued, but you can no longer continue to do what you are doing. So, if you wish to stay, sign on the dotted line, and jump through every single hoop we have set up for you, exactly as we say."

Repeated alcohol misuse result in changes to the brain circuitry.[51] We know that left unmanaged or untreated, over time, repeated misuse will progress predictably to problematic use, or for some, a substance use disorder and addiction. It is only reasonable and smart to intervene early. All employees can benefit from education and thoughtful efforts to deal effectively with both risk factors and strengthen protective factors.[52] Protective factors give people the resources and strength to avoid alcohol misuse and include the things that make people generally healthy and happy, such as positive social connections, and a sense of control over one's successes and failures.[53,54,55] The greatest impact can be gained by reducing alcohol misuse among all cops while at the same time supporting efforts for general health and wellbeing.

It is difficult to determine if education efforts prevent officer alcohol misuse or the onset of a substance use disorder. The biggest benefit of education may be that when a crisis occurs the officer will recognize the utter seriousness of their situation, and know where to turn to get help.

Drowning

Fellow cops have used their best instincts to save a problem drinker cop from drowning, both effectively and ineffectively. Historically, at my agency and likely many others, cops have been proud of their decisive action, showing up before a drunk cop or one who is barely sober starts work, with his bags packed, and dragging him off to treatment. Even if that was effective at times, it only came after repeated tosses of a life preserver or stern lectures about staying out of the deep end. It seems ridiculous to point out that officers must be completely sober at work to be safe, effective and maintain public trust (any argument otherwise is not sustainable). The real rock bottom for problem drinkers is death, and drowning men are dangerous and will take others down with them. We can do better. At the very least, we should focus on these three approaches:

1. Develop an effective response to those who ask for help or those forced to get help, including aftercare support. *Save the drowning man who yells for help.*

2. Provide education about misuse. *Teach everyone to swim or at least how to stay out of the deep end when they do drink.* And only then,

3. Look for problem drinkers. *Start patrolling the pool and beaches looking and listening for trouble.*

Lifeguard work takes skill and training and should not be done by amateurs. Substance misuse and substance use disorders can be very complex and require expert help. Yet when it comes to our coworkers, we tend to want to handle it ourselves, ignore the early signs, symptoms, and prompts and wait until it gets really bad before we take action.

The unfortunate paradox is this, if you seek help you might be considered unsafe or unhealthy, and if you do not seek help you are erroneously considered safe or healthy. Agency progress would be to normalize and elevate the idea of seeking help.

So, we would do well to attend to the police culture. Where I work some cops complain that we do not hang out like we use to, gathering and drinking after work, and they rightfully miss the bonding. It was a lot of fun to gather, laugh and talk about the day, have some drinks and maybe shoot off a round or two. It also functioned as a way to establish who to trust and who was not above reproach. But the bonds dependent on drinking together come with a set of hazards as well. And the bonds may be remarkably fragile, or as one cop told me, "When I got in trouble, those who I thought were my friends didn't give a fuck about me." Between working, carousing and getting some sleep, who is going without? The family. Knowing this, some cops decline, saying, "I gotta go home to get up early with the kids."

Steps in Early Intervention

At a small agency you might be able to ignore drinking problems, statistically, it may not be an issue. Even larger agencies can play the odds, ignore the obvious and hope nothing bad happens. We do this with other things in police work, and the behavior can be reinforced by random success. I think of problems like alcohol misuse or any serious neglect of mental health and wellbeing, kind of like Minnesota and snow. In Minnesota, there is a huge investment by cities, counties and the state in snow plowing, because we know it will pile up and make life difficult or impossible if we do not deal with it. And we get good at dealing with it from repeated direct experience.

Talking to new recruits in the academy about the *evils of alcohol* (education about misuse) would be a huge step at some agencies in that they acknowledge the problem exists and warn officers about it. But there needs to be some response between that minimal education effort and simply waiting to clean up the debris after a senior cop crashes and burns, gets jailed, fired or dies. Early intervention is the necessary addition between these two extremes.

Screening for Problems

Screening for substance misuse can take a number of forms, including private on-line self-assessments. The results of an honest assessment of drinking behavior can result in recommended changes or treatments that can range from relatively minor to major, depending on a number of factors. It is not uncommon for me to be approached by an officer who has done her own on-line assessment and contacts me for further help based on the results. Although this may feel like a dramatic admission to them, I think of it as very ordinary and a sign of good self-care. I refer them to a trained professional who can make a diagnosis and develop a treatment plan as appropriate. All of which remains in the officer's complete control. Ideally, every officer would be confidentially screened for alcohol misuse as they are for any health concern. This could be part of annual reviews, physical fitness assessments or when alerted as part of an Early Intervention System.

Once the screening is complete, the counselor will determine the best course of follow-up action. This may include:

Brief Intervention Depending on the results of a screening, or as part of general health and wellness recommendations, an officer can compare their level of use to safe limits. Additionally, they can be advised on how best to manage behavior and promote healthy decision-making.

Referral to Treatment When Necessary Because some drinking behavior meets the criteria for an alcohol use disorder, and if other interventions have not resulted in any improvement, specialized treatment may be necessary. Those unwilling to engage in professional treatment, can be advised on ways to reduce the risks and harms of ongoing alcohol misuse.[56]

Bad Good Reasons for Not Seeking Treatment

Alcohol use disorder is a disease best treated by skilled professionals. Cops can cite all kinds of "good" reasons to avoid professional help, including: I can't be understood; I need to be treated special because I'm a cop; Treatment is risky to my career or off-duty/overtime earning potential. Or, without evidence, they may conveniently claim the Employee Assistance Program cannot be trusted. This can be a stubborn list, the longer something goes untreated, the harder it is to treat. As serious problems continue untreated, we can do a lot of harm to our loved ones, friends, and our good standing at work. Many who finally get help only wish they had sought it earlier.

Supervisor's Role

Protect the Organism

Although we recognize substance use disorders as an illness, this does not relieve those suffering from it from personal responsibility, and an agency has a responsibility to protect itself. The workplace is like a living organism, which needs protection both from the addicted cop, and for the earnest employee. Earnest employees are those that show up on time, do not ask for special favors and are constant contributors dutifully getting the work done. It is a great disservice to underserve those earnest employees. As a supervisor, you owe it to the earnest, non-addicted employee to make work more sane. There is a logic to this, troubled employees can consume an enormous amount of supervisory attention. Let us say troubled employees are 10% of the work group, many are content to be underperformers and even with your best efforts you will be lucky to get them to budge a quarter-inch. Is this a good use of your time and energy that could be better used to support the other 90%? My analysis is obviously unscientific and I understand that the 10% can create a lot of trouble and liability, but the point is, do not let the chronically lousy worker cause further damage by distracting you from all the rest. There is a chance that as you elevate the workgroup by supporting the good work, the inferior worker's lackluster performance will become more conspicuous and unattractive to the inferior worker.

If we get this backwards, if we are confused about what work is, predictably, we will have big problems. Two things will make the workplace feel crazy, one has to do with all workers, the other with the addicted worker:

- Letting work be about the worker, not about the work that must be done, or

- Letting the addicted people among us define reality.

All workers need to adapt to the work that needs to be done, not the other way around. Too often, workers are allowed to decide if the work tasks suit them or not. When I was a paramedic, I used to joke, "This job would be a lot more fun if it weren't for all these sick and injured people calling for help all the time." The addict will cannibalize a workgroup in pursuit of their often insatiable and shifting needs. We might ask, Is this worker self-centered? Maybe, we all need leadership to lift our head up to a purpose beyond ourselves. Is the addict weak and of poor character? Not necessarily, they may be terrified that this disease has a hold of them; they too are trying to survive.

Some addicted cops are skilled and practiced in not calling attention to themselves. Others have behavior that continually disrupts or causes worry and concern. With the later, I see a parallel between the workplace and the television-style family intervention. This intervention being where the addict's loved ones and a professional gather to confront the addict. The intervention process requires clarifying expectations and boundaries, setting limits. Even if the intervention "fails," in that the addict rejects the process, curses everyone and bursts from the room, all progress is not lost, because those left behind have empowered themselves with the sanity that comes from clarifying expectations and setting boundaries. The organism, whether it is a family or workplace, feels more manageable without the addict in charge.

Those That Seek Help

An agency must first be prepared with an effective response to those seeking help or those forced to get help. This requires first, an acknowledgment of the problem and an intent to act on it, and secondly, planning and forethought. Much of this responsibility can be on the direct supervisor. Every worker can benefit from education, screening and early intervention about alcohol misuse and substance use disorders. But *seeking out* problem drinkers may not only be inappropriate and counterproductive, but also premature when we lack the fundamentals of effective help for those who ask for help. This is not to say that problem drinkers can only be helped if they really want it, or only after they "hit rock bottom," but it is a misplaced effort if it is not part of a comprehensive plan.

Message

Many workplaces, and individuals living well in sobriety, can credit or feel indebted to a single crusader or uncompromising group who, with good hearts, delivered the message of recovery and with hard-won experience helped others in their darkest hours fight the good fight for sobriety. But the problem of substance misuse and disorder is too complex, common, and harmful to the organization to simply rely on motivated individuals. Those that need help are not all in crisis or require treatment. An effective response must be systematic, deliberate, and range from education for all, access to resources, and on-going support. The agency leaders must state their intent up front and consistently apply rules and expectations. The message of recovery, and the hazards of continuing alcohol misuse, is a tough message for a tough audience, but the need is great. Good help can come in many forms, but for a systematic approach, good supervision is the critical link. The police culture has normalized drinking, what is needed is early intervention and to normalize getting help for those with problem drinking. Everyone benefits from being more open about the problem, talking about it, reducing the shame and secrecy associated with it.

"Caring" about Your Cops

We sometimes get confused and think caring for our workers equals only kindness or understanding. Kindness without resolve can be weak. Addicts can chew up and spit out kindness. For the addicted cop, their first love (alcohol) is not the work or anyone there. Expect to be manipulated if you stand between them and their first love. A supervisor must be careful that actions or inactions intended to protect an officer do not cause more trouble for the addicted cop.

I am not suggesting that you need not care about your employee, subordinate or coworker. My intention is to say, be compassionate *and* effective, and if you had to choose one, I would choose being effective. We can care deeply about our coworkers, but as a boss or in some cases, senior officer, it is our job to maintain an orderly work environment. Troubled cops do not need disorder in both their personal *and* work life.

A supervisor can care deeply about the wellbeing of a distressed worker, but that should not be misconstrued to mean they can violate boundaries or forgo their supervisory responsibility to all workers. Non-troubled workers have the right to expect the supervisor will not be overly distracted by the needs or antics of the distressed worker.

If alcohol use disorders are a progressive disease, that means mild can progress to moderate, and moderate to severe. If untreated, severe substance use will result in death, which makes good supervision potentially lifesaving. Effective supervision, which is deliberate and predictable, is caring for your employees, both the addict and the rank and file.

Boundaries and the Helper

When an officer is in distress and someone wishes to help them, the boundaries and rules of engagement differ depending on whom that helper is. One group is concerned friends and family members, another group are police supervisors, command staff or administrators, including human resource personnel. For ease, let us call this second group supervisors. While supervisors must stay focused on work expectations and remain very careful about overstepping personal and professional boundaries, friends, family and coworker friends can play by different rules and may impose themselves in ways that supervisors should not or could not.

Friends and family, and maybe even work buddies, can have special access to the troubled cop due to different boundaries. Friends can show up at the cop's house unannounced, call the cop's spouse or parents, they can talk with them about vague or personal concerns, etc. However, friends and family might also be prone to emotional entanglement.

By contrast, the supervisor's role is based on hierarchy and should pertain to the work. They benefit from being able to view the situation from a healthy distance and take advantage of privileges and responsibilities others do not have, such as work performance data and noticing behavior changes. Precisely because they are not friend or family, the supervisor may be the ideal person to confront a drinking problem. Especially if they understand that their role is not to diagnose the disease, but instead to just address work behavior concerns. The supervisor's duty becomes clearer, less muddled when you know the following three bright-line rules: 1) It is about the work, 2) Stay out of their personal life, and

3) You cannot make them stop, but you can discipline them for not meeting work expectations.

It is the supervisor's responsibility to help maintain a stable work environment where boundaries are respected. All workers, even those who are distressed, benefit from and have the right to show up at work, meet work expectation (even minimally), and leave at the end of the day. In fact, a distressed worker retains the right to self-destruct in their private lives if they wish. Consider consulting human resource staff for any needed clarification about what you can and cannot say and do.

Our Good Feeling

Both the head and the heart are useful if we recognize their limits. A deep good feeling can be our guide, but we might be suspicious of shallow, short-term good feelings and our tendency to confuse the avoidance of discomfort with feeling good.

For many supervisors, their go-to move is the *Come-to-Jesus Speech.* They proudly take the troubled cop aside and give them a stern and impassioned speech about how this is the absolute last time for "this or that bad behavior." Afterwards, the supervisor feels good and, in that moment, the troubled cop may be a convert, but ten minutes later the disease is in charge again. Words mean little, it is actions that matter. It does not make the troubled cop a liar because he breaks the promise. Maybe in that moment they both were of one mind, but ultimately the grasp of the disease is too much. Successful alcohol treatment requires more than willpower. Agencies are ineffective because they either do not act, or they do the wrong thing, because they are unsure what to do or how to do it, or consciously chose the easiest path.

Bright-Line Rules

What qualifies many cops that become supervisors and managers is the simple fact that they are promoted. These supervisors essentially have to survive on their wits, untrained and unprepared, and probably take their lead from what they have observed being supervised and managed. When I was newly promoted, I was fortunate to hear a retired public works manager named Milan Mockovak speak. I took his central message to be, "It's about the work." The focus of worker efforts and supervision of workers must be on the work that must be done, not on the peripheral issues. I was additionally relieved when he warned us to stay out of people's personal lives.[57] It seems obvious now, but just months earlier I had been a patrol cop with the mistaken belief that a good supervisor should "care" about his cops but I had no clear understanding of the boundaries.

Whereas personal or non-work issues are limitless, work expectations are definable and within the grasp of supervision. If something is not working, it might not be because we are not doing enough of it, it might be because we are doing too much.

Work is about the work — focus on work behavior. If failure to meet work expectations or some specific action or inaction has gotten the supervisor's attention, clearly defined work rules and expectations should be used to correct them. Otherwise, leave them alone.

Stay out of their personal life. People have a right to not function well in their personal lives. Even troubled employees should expect supervisors to leave them alone and stay out of their personal lives. The boss has a right, and may be well advised, to keep the relationship about the work. For the supervisor, being invited into a cop's personal life can be a form of manipulation. This can be extremely difficult in police work, in part because we promote from within, and coworkers can become supervisors. But just understanding this dynamic can help get your mind right.

Ideally, workers are constant contributors who make personal and professional progress year after year. However, I respect the fact that some people are just trying to maintain as they struggle with personal problems. In a long career, people should be permitted to move in and out of three categories of functionality, doing well, doing poorly, and just maintaining. For some, "progress" means not going backwards, and they may need a period where they "fake" their wellbeing as they work on their issues privately as is their right to a point. That point being, again, meeting work expectations. Good supervision should recognize all three types of functionality. Further inquiry of what a supervisor notices may be warranted, but the right to say "Thanks, but no thanks," belongs to the worker.

The idea of someone being a "functional" alcoholic may be a myth. They may show up at work or at home but showing up may not be enough. But the concept that an employee has a right to not function well away from the job is helpful for the supervisor by organizing their thinking, to include: a) what is my role, b) what are work expectations, c) what are the limits to my responsibility.

You cannot make them get treatment. No person can make someone else get sober or successfully complete treatment; the supervisor can't, EAP director can't, the chief of police, sheriff or warden can't. But the chief, sheriff or warden can fire them for failing to meet properly documented work expectations. Or make keeping their job contingent on successfully completing treatment and aftercare. Meeting or not meeting work expectations is really the only leverage an administration has. There are cops among us that would still be addicted or dead if they had not been required to randomly do piss tests. A paramedic acquaintance told me, with no bitterness, that his bosses did everything they could for him, but it took getting fired for him to get sober. Not everyone gets to keep his or her job. Combined with an effective assessment, treatment and aftercare program, we can use this leverage to our advantage. Ultimately it is the individual cop's responsibility to remain fit for duty, but if drinking problems at a particular agency routinely cause cops to lose their jobs, it is a failure of imagination, planning and prioritizing on the part of the agency.

But you can make treatment look very desirable. One of the advantages in police work is the fact that alcohol misuse *can* cost a cop his job. Having a cop fear that the department will take his gun and badge away is a great motivator and a kind of leverage the general public may not have.

Similarly, pilots who have alcohol addictions fear losing his or her wings. In fact, pilots have had an industry-specific treatment option for decades. One of the most successful rehab programs ever is the Human Intervention Motivation Study (HIMS). Under the program there are over 13,000 pilots flying with a special medical license for addiction. Since the mid-1970, 6000 pilots have been treated and returned to the cockpit. Members of the public are three times more likely to relapse than a pilot. The science-based HIMS program is threefold:

- FAA-approved treatment facility,

- Monitoring, and drug testing, and

- If cleared to fly, ongoing treatment for at least 3 years.[58]

Taking Action

The days of fellow cops' informal "ambush" before roll call to escort a colleague to treatment are generally over. With nothing equivalent or better to take their place, some agencies essentially ignore problems so long that a troubled cop eventually fires himself. A lack of supervisor training, support and a good plan enable the avoidance of problems. Despite this, an individual supervisor with a clear sense of purpose and responsibility can still find a way to do the right thing. A supervisor, unclear about his purpose and function, will do the wrong thing.

A good example of the wrong thing is when an absent worker is marked as leave-no-pay, meaning they have run out of sick time and vacation and they are given a pass instead of discipline. This act by the supervisor is crossing an otherwise clear line of demarcation and in effect makes showing up or not for work arbitrary. The supervisor is actively ignoring a problem and his internal message may be that he does not know for sure if the cop has a drinking problem, or the problem has not yet reached a level where it is his business or responsibility to act. This may be part of a misguided effort to protect the officer. Yet the real reason the supervisor fails to act correctly is more likely because it is a difficult situation, and he does not know what to do.

It is never the supervisor's job to diagnose the disease; it is not necessarily the supervisor's responsibility to discover or expose the alcohol or drug problem. His responsibility is to act on unmet work expectations or policy violations. Sometimes that action is corrective, discipline, or further investigation. Inaction is, in effect, an action, and the supervisor must know that everyone is watching.

Reasons to take action can be obvious, such as an off-duty arrest, suspected on-duty intoxication, and the not so obvious behavior such as noticing that an officer avoids all supervisory contact. Sometimes others alert the supervisor to worrisome behavior, appearance changes or strained work relationships. Compelled supervisory action could result from activation of an Early Intervention System, via sick time usage, internal affairs complaints, squad crashes, or other preset indicators.

A series of prompts can assist the supervisor in determining when to take action. The U.S. Office of Personnel Management publication *Alcoholism in the Workplace: A Handbook for Supervisors* lists the following signs to look for which all seem applicable for police officers.

> *Leave and Attendance problems:* unexplained or unauthorized absences from work, frequent tardiness, Monday or Friday absences, frequent unplanned absences due to "emergencies" (e.g. household repairs, car trouble, family emergencies, legal problems).

> *Performance problems:* missed deadlines, careless or sloppy work or incomplete assignments, production quotas not met, many excuses for incomplete assignments or missed deadlines, faulty analysis.

> *Relationships at Work:* relationships with coworkers may become strained, employee may be belligerent, argumentative, or short-tempered, especially in the mornings or after weekends or holidays, employee may become a "loner."[59]

Supervisor's Action Plan for Success

Help Yourself First

To get right-minded about our purpose and function when it comes to helping a troubled employee or coworker, it is most useful to look at ourselves and understand why we might be tempted to take less effective short cuts. We are generally unskilled, unpracticed, and untrained in this form of intervention. It can be extremely uncomfortable to make demands about work expectations or ask a cop direct questions about observed or suspected problems. Some of us would rather be the first through a doorway on a weapons call than wrongly accuse a coworker or see a cop cry.

The core of the problem might be that it is hard, and we understand their suffering and want to protect them. Cops with alcohol use disorders may have diminished decision-making abilities, not completely dissimilar to an adolescent. If they think otherwise, they may need to be reminded that their best thinking got them into this mess, and they may need to trust someone else's thinking for a bit. This makes good leadership critical, a kind of detached parenting or what has been called "tough love," to help them survive or find their better selves. They need clear direction and maybe kindness, but sympathy may be the last thing they need. Above all, they need the helper to be clear minded.

Some self-awareness about our vulnerability is precisely why we must be more intentional and deliberate when we see one of our own suffering. In order to be truly effective, we must turn down emotion, and turn up rational thought. Our tendency to do what makes us feel better in difficult situations can lead to actions that are very misguided. This might be called co-dependence, enabling, or caretaking. If our actions are shortsighted, they may delay natural consequences, and in some cases, the troubled person would be better off without us. Just as families may "love an addict to death," supervisors can prolong suffering by either inaction or enabling. The enabling can remove some of the discomfort that would otherwise force people to deal with the consequences of their behavior. For the addict, things need to stay uncomfortable.

1. Take the First Step

Consider what you are dealing with. If the officer has an alcohol use disorder, a progressive brain disease, it not only affects her decision-making, but makes her very skilled and highly motivated to protect her secret. She can be like a shape-shifter and extremely hard to pin down.

Continued alcohol use feels essential to her survival. She also may be afraid and ashamed that this disease has a hold of her, despite her best efforts to control it. Others may be deep in denial and willfully ignorant of the consequences of their behavior. Some simply are not ready to self-reflect or make meaningful changes. Thus, if you naively enter their world without a plan or preparation, you only risk doing more harm, and if you try to get between them and their first love, you will fail. Your role is not to diagnose, prove addiction, or catch them in a lie; your role is to address specific work expectations, express concerns, offer resources, and follow-up on any required action.

If the specific topic of alcohol misuse is addressed, ask them if they can identify negative consequences of that use. It is possible the cop will confess that they are a miserable wretch, owe their life to you and commit on the spot to whatever needs to be done, but that is not likely. You will be most effective if you have already established yourself as trustworthy and forthright, but even if this is someone you only casually know, you are establishing a relationship, beginning a process, not swinging for a home run.

2. Plan Ahead

The following is a guide when prompted to take action, for example, you have reason to believe an officer is a problem drinker, and it has negatively impacted their work. You may never feel fully prepared to confront a tough issue, but you can advantage yourself in many ways.

Find a Point Person. Identify and get commitment from a point person. Whether it is you or another supervisor, someone must take the lead, take ownership of the plan and process.

Pursue Buy-In. You need buy-in from key people to establish a unified front. This may be your boss and co-supervisors. It may not be necessary to describe the source of your concerns, but if you are making new demands of a subordinate, you must communicate and coordinate your plan with these people to avoid an end-around and sergeant shopping. Instinctually, the troubled cop will look for the weak link. The idea is to design success and build your own network of support and to avoid failure due to inattention or a porous front line. Beware: A lack of buy-in can be a product of a fellow supervisor's own problem with alcohol, making them uncooperative, subversive or unable to be provide clearheaded support.

Gather facts. Expect your facts to be challenged and know that not being able to substantiate your assertions will be deflating, a distraction and derail any progress. You need not feel that you are building a case against the person or trying to diagnose or prove a drinking problem. Instead, you are pointing out specific work expectations and how compliance will be monitored. Observations about these expectations should be specific, objective and timely.

3. Take Action

If you have given thought to what you are dealing with, and done appropriate planning, you will be able to take the action step with more confidence.

The Serious Talk. Taking action on these concerns requires a meeting with the troubled cop. This meeting requires planning, preparation and practice. When I was a new patrol supervisor I became aware of some troubling officer behavior, I thought, "Oh hell no, not on my watch." So, I called the officer in for a talk. He promptly placed a tape recorder on the desk between us. I lost my nerve and the recording I am sure included several minutes of me babbling. My lack of experience, preparation and planning made me not only ineffective, but also counterproductive.

You need to know what you are up against. By the time a drinking problem gets your attention, you must know it has likely have been going on for a very long time, and the troubled cop is way ahead of you on deflecting concern.

Meet privately. The meeting should be free of distractions and diversions. Ideally, attendees will be freed from the divided attention that comes with having to monitor the radio or other obligations. You must allow enough time to avoid the temptation for either of you to try to escape when things get predictably uncomfortable.

Stay with the Plan. It is your job to manage the meeting. Keep your empathy or sympathy in check; otherwise you can lose your objectivity. State your concerns, ask your questions, and make specific factual observations. Avoid debate. Clarity becomes pivotal and requires both thoughtful statements and good listening. In some cases, a contract of sorts or progress improvement plan defining expectations may be required.

Not all careers can be saved, and willingness to do so at all costs is a management failure. We can inform, encourage, remind and demand that workers meet work expectations, but ultimately it is their responsibility. We cannot fix their health and personal problems, but we can offer expert help and if they are willing, assist in the necessary steps to obtain it.

Find Your Resolve. Much like the street, where crooks, addicts, and ne'er-do-wells test your resolve, the addicted cop will look for cracks in your armor. It is useful to recognize his fear may drive a lot of his hostile or anti-social behavior at this point. It must be very frightening to lose control to drugs or alcohol. He may be experiencing powerlessness over an addiction and his life has become unmanageable, and this can make him desperate. It is essential that you fortify yourself against pushback and diversions. Without resolve and forethought, you may stumble badly when confronted by hostile counter accusations and distractions like, "Why are you picking on me?" or "What about this other guy or that other event?"

Much like the noise complaint while on patrol, we are not picking on them at random. They got our attention by one way or another, and we intend to deal with it. Be deliberate, calm, and stay with the plan, hold the line.

As time goes on, pushback can be viewed as a positive sign that the point person is successfully holding the troubled employee accountable. In the short term it is easier to ignore problems. Taking supervisory action at first is more work, but eventually should become easier or at least somewhat clear. You know you are on the right track when things eventually become harder for them and easier for you.

Express Confidence. It is tempting to view the troubled cop as *the problem*, each of you staking your claim while (literally or figuratively) seated across from each other on opposite sides of a table. It may not be about being tough, though it could be if tough means stating clear expectations and holding to them. Instead, you may consider imagining that you are both on the same side of the table, together viewing the problem before you. Make it less personal and more performance.

Your role can be to help her see the problem and the way out. Express confidence in her ability to overcome difficulties, as she has done before. It may feel like it makes sense to effectively say, "I got my eye on you, don't f-up." But most cops I know want to succeed and a little external confidence can help. So, a better approach can be, "I know you are going through a rough spot, I want you to succeed, let's come up with a plan and meet regularly over the next couple of weeks to check-in."

If you get your mind right and approach the meeting with forethought and your own network of support, you may hear yourself saying things like, "You can't keep doing what you are doing...acting like you are acting...but we don't want to lose you. So, the following is what I am asking you to agree to..." Troubled cops do not soon forget the straight talk given with genuine concern. But success is fact based and dependent on their actions, not promises. Addicted people understand consequences. Whether it is social, legal or occupational, consequences get people sober.

It is about the work, and the Serenity Prayer *(God, grant me the serenity to accept the things I cannot change, courage to change the things I can, and the wisdom to know the difference)* can apply to the supervisor too. You cannot make them get treatment, but you can discipline them, you cannot discipline them unless you document failure to comply with rules. You cannot do any of this without a plan.

Arrange for Professional Involvement. If an officer is agreeable to getting help with alcohol misuse, the next step is a professional assessment. A diagnosis of alcohol use disorder may be mild, moderate or severe. Severe cases or those complicated with co-occurring problems such as depression or increased suicide risk may require immediate hospitalization or admission to a treatment facility that includes detoxification (for stabilization and withdrawal management).

We fail to effectively supervise, not because we do not care, but more often because of a lack of skill and experience, being wrong-minded about alcohol misuse and use disorders. Our attempts to intervene can be ineffective or make things worse because we do not act or do the wrong thing, often with the best of intentions. We need our organization to function well; to be organized and approach problems systematically and with forethought; and to have a plan that is supported at multiple levels. Most importantly, you need to get your thinking right: about the officer, the workplace, your role as helper, and the disease.

CHAPTER 9

STRUGGLE AND CHANGE
And Live Another Day

Struggle

When my children were toddlers, my wife helped me see that they became extra crabby and irritable just before a big change, for example, taking their first steps. With this insight, I found it easy to imagine that their rapidly developing brain was ready to walk, but their body or body-brain connection was not.

We have accomplished great things when you consider we start out completely dependent on another for our own survival. As children, we may have imagined that being an adult means you arrive at some steady or stable place, that change is over. But as adults, we realize we take little steps, or big steps, our whole life. And yet we never really arrive, and we can never return, and unless we are preparing to die, we just keep moving forward. There is no static or steady state, left unattended, things moves from a state of order to disorder. It takes energy and effort to not slip into disorder. To be disillusioned means you have rid yourself of an illusion, which is a good thing—a good thing that may feel bad. This sounds troublesome, bleak, nightmarish maybe, or at least tiresome and disillusioning, but it might be a matter of correcting our thinking. This constant change actually means we are not done yet.

The Harvard Happiness study showed that the role of genetics proved less important to a person's longevity than the person's level of satisfaction with relationships in midlife, which is now recognized as a good predictor of healthy aging. The research also debunked the idea that people's personalities are "set like plaster" by age 30 and cannot be changed. "Those who were clearly train wrecks when they were in their 20's or 25's turned out to be wonderful octogenarians," said psychiatrist and researcher George Vaillant. "On the other hand, alcoholism and major depression could take people who started life as stars and leave them at the end of their lives as train wrecks."[1]

At times, things come easy as if you have the wind at your back; other times things are a struggle. When you consider your greatest growth, it was likely during the struggle. The easy times are a time to rest and recover while awaiting the next challenge.

Sometimes we struggle because of unreasonable expectations. I once heard a group of immigrants describing Americans as having this strange outlook, expecting life to be hardship-free. By comparison, they expected a certain amount of life trouble. When things were good, they enjoyed the blessing, and when things were bad, they endured until things got better. All without the extra burden of believing, "The universe is picking on me." They seemed happier. I heard a version of this while working with a Viet Nam vet who would say any time something was difficult or disappointing, "Well, at least it's not raining and nobody is shooting at us."

And although tranquility is not a "fixed" state either, we can cultivate longer periods of it where we have fewer highs and lows, or highs that are not too high and lows that are not too low. Some amount of personal struggle is unavoidable, some is absolutely necessary for growth, and I cannot easily imagine a time when this will not be so. Unease and distress can be reframed as an indication that a change is needed or you are on the right track and a change is coming.

Do or Die

Toughness has a lot to do with how well we struggle or how we view hardship itself. I once heard the great author and historian Studs Terkel speak; he was best known for his oral histories of common Americans. He compared two men during the Great Depression who both had beans for dinner. The one accustomed to steak complained bitterly and was disheartened; the other, accustomed to beans, was satisfied to have something to eat. Resiliency is knowing that beans will sustain you, and that you can survive on them longer than you think. The strongest among us have endured or overcome, but maybe kept these achievements to themselves, a shadow resume of sorts.

Complete freedom, being totally unbound does not exist and seeking it is foolhardy and undisciplined. As Winston Churchill said, "It's not enough that we do our best; sometimes we have to do what's required."[2] When I taught high school for a short period, a student told me that his parents expressed complete trust in him, that everything he did was fine. This was highly distressing to him; he felt rudderless. Boundaries, or having something to push against, paradoxically gives us more freedom, not less. We *do*, by way of struggle, hardship and efforts to change and improve ourselves, or we *die* by way of entropy.

Even if we were to find a script on how to live our lives, we have to figure out much of it on our own. Listening to our parents could save us a lot of trouble, but we seem to have to learn things the hard way. Benjamin Franklin had a plan of sorts for himself, but he was not born with it. He wrote it himself, inspired by a bible verse. Franklin's 13 virtues were a lifelong pursuit that in totality could be described as a disciplined life. You may view hardships as a challenge or opportunity to practice virtues, not something to be eliminated. As some have said, "The more I practice, the luckier I get."[3] With practice what we eventually achieve is a disciplined mind, which directs all other behavior.

The Good Struggle

In grade school, I had good reason to believe that I was dumb because I had an undiagnosed reading problem, but fortunately for me it never occurred to me that I was dumb. I also recognized the system was broken, often the teacher was lazy and unskilled. I recall the math teacher stating a problem, the smartest kid in the room would shout out the answer, and we would move on to the next problem, useless. My reading problem profoundly affected my day-to-day functioning, but only strengthened my diligence and perseverance.

In 1979 Jim Stigler, a graduate student, went to Japan to research teaching methods. In a 2012 NPR broadcast he told of being in the back row of a crowded fourth-grade math class where he watched the teacher teach the class how to draw three-dimensional cubes on paper. Stigler explains, "and one kid was just totally having trouble with it. His cube looked all cockeyed, so the teacher said to him, 'Why don't you go put yours on the board?' So right there I thought, 'That's interesting! He took the one who can't do it and told him to go and put it on the board.'"

Stigler knew that in American classrooms it was usually the smartest or most eager kid who would be invited to the board. He described watching with interest and trepidation as the Japanese student came to the board and started drawing. Still, the cube looked wrong. Every so often the teacher would ask the class if the kid had gotten it right, and they would look up from their work, and shake their heads no. Stigler said, "I realized that I was sitting there starting to perspire," he continued, "because I was really empathizing with this kid. I thought, 'This kid is going to break into tears!'" Despite what Stigler thought was a very difficult situation, the kid remained composed and continued to draw the cube. "And at the end of the class, he did make his cube look right! And the teacher said to the class, 'How does that look, class?' And they all looked up and said, 'He did it!' And they broke into applause. The kid smiled a huge smile and sat down, clearly proud of himself."[4]

Stigler went on to describe how he and his colleagues did a study of first-grade students. "We decided to go out and give the students an impossible math problem to work on, and then we would measure how long they worked on it before they gave up." The American students "worked on it less than 30 seconds on average and then they basically looked at us and said, 'We haven't had this.' But the Japanese students worked for the entire hour. And finally, we had to stop the session because the hour was up." Stigler wondered aloud what a big difference that kind of behavior could have spread over a lifeitme.[5]

In the animal world, it is all about survival. A YouTube video titled, "Mama Polar Bear Saves Her Little Cub Who Can't Swim Yet" concludes with the adult bear running to the cub's aid and scooping the cub out of the water. What was most fascinating was how long the adult bear watched the cub struggle from a distance and only sprang into action when the cub had reached some level of danger, but not before.

Everyone Struggles

As the EAP guy for the police department, I make an effort to see and be seen. When making my rounds through the police department I sometimes get *The Look* from someone. I interpret it, remarkably reliably it turns out, as "Can he see how much I am suffering?" People who know me will ask? "How is EAP going?" My answer, "I *think* it's going okay." Emphasizing my doubt, not so much superstition, but I know so much pain and suffering is hidden that I do not want to be overconfident. There have been days where I am overtaxed or not fully recovered from vicarious trauma, so I avoid the rounds for fear of getting *The Look* and not having anything to give.

Being that I am not a therapist, I try to stay where I belong in the therapeutic process, which is in the areas of permission, education and support. I want people who are feeling troubled to come my way. A common introductory comment from cops is "I was going to call you." I see a big part of my role as giving people permission to feel bad and encouragement that they are not alone. I know that we can feel ashamed and afraid of the darkness within. Hank Williams captured this in the song, "I'm So Lonesome I Could Cry".[6]

In an interview, Williams was pressed to answer where the lyrics came from. He responded, "Everybody has a little darkness in them. They may not like it, may not want to know about it, but it's there. And I show it to them." The suffering Williams sings about is universal, and we find solace and consolation in great art because it brings us together, because it reminds us that we are all the same. We all suffer in the same way.[7]

The Right Struggle

Health and disease commingle throughout life. Our response to difficulty can be healthy or unhealthy, adaptive or maladaptive. More likely, it is somewhere in between, a jumbled mix of both. Either way, it is all coping. Health and disease are on a continuum, not an all-or-none thing. And we are, as people in recovery like to express it, "not bad people trying to get good, but sick people getting better."

That is why I know that when a cop shares his suffering with me, the act of sharing a hidden pain can feel like a sacred space, because for some, this may be the first time ever he has expressed to someone an inner darkness we all share. We can become afraid of our intense feelings and painful thoughts.

Quite possibly, the cost of a big thinking brain, the human brain, is some amount of anxiety and depression. But that same brain can reflect on itself. We can observe our own thinking, practice managing our thoughts and feelings, at the very least ask ourselves, "Is what I'm thinking factually true?" It is like capturing a thought in its infancy and directing it toward the best-case scenario or the most realistic or most likely outcome, rather than focusing on the worst or less likely case. We can also pause and acknowledge an uncomfortable thought or feeling, even if it frightens us. We may fear that acknowledging them will make them more real or that they will never go away, but the paradox is that some unpleasant thoughts and feelings may just need to have their say, to be fully experienced, not pushed aside or avoided. They can be remarkably persistent for our own good, so pausing to acknowledge them may be great progress for some.

Being honest with yourself, and in some cases with others, can be transformative. Healing, and real and necessary change, can only occur in truthful environments. At the very least it is efficient in that you put your energies toward the real or core issues, rather than superficial or misguided causes. Everyone struggles, and it can feel shameful and lonely, but humans have more in common than we have different, and the issues we struggle with often are around sometimes common themes.

A Crisis is a Terrible Thing to Waste

Mental and emotional distress can be our friend, but unfortunately as we look for the quickest relief, we may squander it. There have been times when a distressed cop is talking to me, and I have to suppress a smile because I am so pleased he is asking for help or sharing his suffering, which puts him on the verge of transformation. Carl Jung, the brilliant psychiatrist, congratulated people in crisis. He told them they had been given a chance for necessary growth as he had knowledge that we all want different things at different times of our life. There is a need for continuous adjustment. Jung described the gradual emergence of the true self through balancing or integrating conflicting parts of the personality, including those parts that previously had been neglected. People who avoid this transition and do not reorient their lives appropriately miss the chance for psychological growth.[8]

In many cases it is probably naive, or at least inaccurate, to think that it is one bad thing causing suffering and one fix to make us better. It is probably human nature to let some things get to a crisis point before we make a change or take action. A crisis can force us out of autopilot. When a big unwanted problem arrives, we become disoriented, and it can force us deeper. I have heard it described this way: in moments of suffering we discover that we are more than who we thought we were, we discover our basement and the basement below that.[9]

The Good Discomfort

Our unavoidable personal struggles, like a recurring bad dream, return again and again until we get the message. Or like a fussy infant, they persist until we attend to the need. Facing our troubles and fears is the opposite of avoiding. When these difficulties come into our consciousness or are realized in our bodies, sometimes this alone is transformative. It is always a chance to practice new skills, new ways of thinking, new ways of interacting with others and ourselves. Paradoxically, those who avoid discomfort are more likely to be uncomfortable than those who periodically embrace discomfort. Fortitude and toughness have a lot to do with being comfortable with discomfort.

Bad is Good

Some things turn out to be upside-down and backwards, including our thinking or the messages we get from others. It takes a different point of view to see what is real or to end up eventually being thankful for a hardship. Because something feels bad, or is uncomfortable, it is easy to label it as bad; which is sometimes true and keeps us in line, but not always. It turns out we might be stopping progress prematurely because of its related discomfort. Below are uncomfortable thoughts and feelings that may actually be a sign of good things happening or progress:

- Sadness
- Fear
- Irritability
- Anxiety and restlessness
- Confrontational
- Dissatisfaction
- Feeling lost
- Strange and intense dreams
- Questioning your friendships and relationships

You might find it a far better strategy to work to become more comfortable being uncomfortable than trying to avoid discomfort altogether. During times of change, we might wish our lives would return to normal. Sometimes a cop will comment to me that she wishes things would return to the way they were. What she is going through may look like progress to me so I might reply, "You cannot go back because you are a different person from when this started. This suffering has given you something."

Change

Some life changes require a major lifestyle overhaul while others only a small adjustment. Some change results from gaining a different point of view following a sudden insight or prolonged suffering. The exact path or formula is hard to predict. For example, a cop who is prescribed a number of medications and is diagnosed as pre-diabetic, if properly motivated, will have to get a new diet and commit to an exercise routine, an overhaul of some kind. For others, simply becoming aware of a habit or behavior is enough to initiate change. When someone complains about poor posture and theorizes that they need to take yoga classes, another might see the solution as simply standing up straighter. Making plans to change can be a way of putting change off, avoiding it. The phrase or thought, "I'll do it tomorrow" is self-deception-speak for "I'm not gonna do it." Some have discovered that the best way to make a change, or take on a quality you admire, is to act as if you already have it. Some within the addiction recovery community express this as "Fake it until you make it," or as I recall from an episode of the Andy Griffith Show, sheriff Taylor tells Opie, as he leaves for school, "Do a good day's work and act like somebody."

Some changes or self-improvements can appear suddenly, while others require prolonged or ongoing effort; we do not always get to choose, but fundamental to effective change is accurately identifying the real issue. Humans are designed to forget some stuff and not even see other stuff. We have a tendency towards blind spots and self-deception, which may at times be both useful and problematic. When it comes to diet for example, eating less and exercising more may seem obviously necessary, but for some, food can be linked with deep meaning or a sense of deprivation can be a trigger. Self-awareness can both enlighten us to the need for a change and also inform us why it may be difficult. So better posture may just be a matter of a conscious effort to stand up straighter, but it may also be a problem with the spine or a diminished sense of self.

Change can be illusive, so it helps to think of it in terms of daily tasks, bringing it up close to your face. Let inspiration come from the change, not rely on inspiration to produce the change.

Motivation versus Routine

A workshop speaker described a single metal beam bridging the roofs of two skyscrapers and asked the audience if they would cross it. Everyone replied that they would not. He then added that while you were on one rooftop, your toddler was on the other, dangerously close to the edge and in need of saving. Now would you cross it?

Being highly motivated to do something or make a necessary change is very helpful, combine that with good information and resources, and you will probably succeed. Occasionally you hear people use phrases like, "I was sick of feeling sick," or "Do what you've always done, get what you've always gotten." However, motivation can be fickle, unreliable or short-lived, and it does not hold up well to boredom, low self-esteem, high self-esteem, competition for time and any number of things that can be summarized in the phrase, "I don't feel like it."

Getting out of bed and on your feet before consulting your own opinion on whether you want to might be best. Olympic athletes in training hear the messages in their head, "No," "Stop," "Enough already," and their success can be dependent on ignoring these messages. I once heard an underwater breath-holding champion describe how his technique was completely dependent on distracting himself.

Good habits and routines can carry us through. It seems far more effective to rely less on motivation and inspiration, and more on routine, practicing good habits, and a commitment to specific action steps. Focusing on steady progress, instead of bursts of passion.

Make Your Own Luck

Sometimes a "bad" thing can turn out to be a good thing, a blessing of sorts. Hard times, can be a really important turning point in a person's life, but you may never know for sure, especially when you are right in the middle of it. Not only do we need to rethink what is good luck and bad luck, we may adapt what has been said, "Chance favors the prepared mind."[10]

Once, following a guy who was acting suspiciously into a convenience store, I found him hiding in an aisle. I patted him down, walked him outside and ID'd him, without wants or warrants I let him go. What I did not do was search the area where I had found him. If I had, I would have (as the surveillance video showed) found the loaded pistol he ditched as I rounded the aisle. I have always paid close attention to my near misses, at least those that I knew of. I got lucky that time, but luck has little value in police work. When I was a patrolman, I regularly critiqued my own behavior, as a patrol supervisor, it was my job to critique others, and I had no patience for relying on luck and its useless friend wishful thinking. These seem like dangerous shortcuts or laziness, I was not willing to play the odds with my life or others. If I were to take a shortcut, I wanted it to be an informed one, the most direct route based on experience and forethought, having first experienced the long road. This is not to suggest I was not at times lazy or undisciplined, because I was, but if I were, I at least acknowledged it to myself. Making your own luck has nothing to do with luck and everything to do with your own best efforts. And your own best effort can begin immediately, starting with confronting your own self-deception and avoidance of difficult but necessary things, like being more honest with yourself, meeting your responsibilities, and focusing your energies on what is within your control.

Action Not Talk

Sometimes we talk about something we hope to do, like, "I am going to volunteer to be a Big Brother (Big Sister)," but it stops there at just talk. The reward comes with expressing it and the admiration of others for having such an intention. If you seriously want a change, be it to go back to school and finish your degree, or start a side business, or floss your teeth, and if you are going to talk about it, make it a commitment to someone whom you do not want to disappoint. But more importantly, take the next step, set up an appointment at the college or buy dental floss. Most importantly, you want progress, to be somewhere else the next week. When I speak to officers in distress, I like to reassure them with phrases like; "Let's see if we can get you to a better spot, further down the road." Getting better, even just a little better can be very satisfying, self-perpetuating and affirming.

Running and Walking

There is the old phrase, *it is easier to turn a moving ship,* the first step or steps can be the hardest, yet most important to building some momentum. There are two schools of thought regarding making progress and over-coming inertia, and both require looking forward. The first, *keep your eye on the prize.* When I was learning to drive my oldest brother commented that I was jerking the wheel from side to side too much. I was making adjustments for every defect in the road in front of me. He said, "Look farther down the road." I did, and things smoothed out.

The second way of thinking is to focus on what is right in front of you. This seems to contradict the first way, so we can think of this as walking and the previous example of driving as running. Life successes seem more a result of small, but important daily moment-to-moment choices, attending to what is right in front of us, especially when starting out or when things get difficult. "The best place for your focus, it turns out, is something small and real…switch your attention to what's going on in front of you."[11] By dutifully attending to the small things in our life, daily maintenance, from making our bed at the beginning of the day and saying our prayers at the end.

Design Success

Self-improvement is a life-long pursuit requiring daily contributions, sometimes seeking, and sometimes surrendering. When seeking, it is important to be clear-sighted about what you are trying to achieve. The action steps should be realistic and obtainable as if designed for success. There is a lot of bad advice out there, and most of it is free. You get what you pay for, if you want more, you must pay more, payment in the form of your own effort. Much of the work of self-improvement evolves around specific behaviors driven by specific habits. The first step in doing better is to stop doing worse, or indulging a bad habit, then occupy yourself with replacing a bad habit with a good one. You can weaken a stubborn bad habit by extending to hours or days the time between its occurrence.

If you really want something, commit to it and persevere, and leave out whether you feel like it or not. Or as one of my friends says, "to succeed, a gap analysis needs to happen. Get a grip on the current situation and make incremental steps to move in the direction you want to go." [12] If it is difficult, you are on the right track, if you want an easier route, save that for an easy problem. Self-improvement is not always about going after what you want, sometimes it involves changing what you want. For example, it can be about wanting less or learning to want what you already have. It is up to you to figure out which is which.

Help from Others

Being just rational or just emotional is dangerously out of balance and does not utilize your full spectrum of human "intelligence" and ability. If you are just strong, you are not fully human. Revealing vulnerability is not without risk, and it can be a signal to others to help or exploit, revealing their character. Cops are good at not retreating and revealing a vulnerability can feel like retreating. But there seems to be this thing in human nature, or the universe, that certain help will not arrive until you are at a level of surrender or honest vulnerability, and that help can come from surprising people and places. It may not be so mysterious if you recognize that at some level, all people know they have a little darkness in them, and it is not until you are wholly dependent on the mercy of others, that the universe steps in.

With a few exceptions, we need each other, we are interdependent. It is natural to struggle and natural to ask for help. It is against our natural human impulse to withhold sharing personal concerns. And it is our better selves that reach out to help others.

Burn the Boat

Some change cannot occur until you fully commit, unable to fail. I was surprised once by what I heard a father tell his young adult child, instead of saying, "No matter what, we are here for you. You always have a home with us," he instead said the opposite, "You must succeed because you are no longer a child. You must make your own home." Whether we operate this way or not, as parents, leaders or with ourselves, it is good to consider our resolve. We know this as cops; those we ask or tell, evaluate our resolve. Do we mean what we say, and say what we mean? We should ask this of ourselves. Some self-improvement requires a seeking, some surrender. Courage is starting the journey without necessarily knowing where it will end. Some self-improvement requires we take a step backwards, and most improvement requires walking or running forward. The common theme in all of these is that rather than do nothing, we move.

Resilience and Attitude

Resilient means strong and flexible, quick to recover, tough, but the word has become so overused and associated with some "vague concept of 'character'"[13] that I was reluctant to mention it in this book. Mental toughness is more of an attitude and set of certain skills that are acquired and can be taught. Building resilience is not all tough guy stuff; it can be both getting thicker skin and a softer heart. It can involve specific learned skills as well as rest and recovery before and after psychological trauma or difficulties. In their book *The Resilience Factor,* authors Karen Reivich and Andrew Shattel describe how resilience is associated with values that suggest a real need for courage and adaptability. Their list of values includes:[14]

- Flexibility/adapting to change

- Thinking styles

- Emotional regulation (emotional intelligence)

- Impulse control

- Empathy

- Optimism

- Self-efficacy

- Reaching out

Your attitude about difficulties is what matters most; the key is how you view bad things (negative life events) as a chance to learn, grow, meet a challenge and adapt, or as personal attacks that are unfair and forever wounding. As we in public safety work rightly acknowledge the potential mental and emotional harm associated with the work, we have been a bit seduced into focusing almost exclusively on our vulnerabilities or susceptibilities, and less on our areas of strength and protective factors. Being well rested, emotionally healthy, having strong and positive family ties and social connections, and having a feeling that one has control over one's successes and failures are all protective factors.

It is natural to identify a harm and look for the cause and what made the recipient vulnerable. But a higher level of thinking, one that is more productive and useful, is to look at protective factors — what makes someone strong and less vulnerable. We can look around at a roll call and see bitter angry cops who are super cynical and eager to engage anyone in a bitch session or to mock anyone with an optimist view, they can get lots of attention. Actually, those cops might be feeling afraid, pessimism may help them feel like they are in the know, not lost in a big scary or disappointing world. But we probably would do well to observe, or at least have some curiosity about, the calm, supportive cop who is eager to go to work.

In a *New Yorker* article titled "How People Learn to Become Resilient" author Maria Konnikova compiles some of the newest thinking on resilience. The article points out that researchers and the common man have figured out that life success is a result of two factors, "individual, psychological factors, and external environmental factors, or disposition on the one hand and luck on the other." [15] We might consider that it mostly comes down to what is within our control, disposition, or our attitude. Even with bad luck, we still only have influence over our response to it, again attitude.

Researcher Emmy Werner studied a group of six hundred and ninety-eight children for thirty-two years and found several elements that predicted resilience. "A resilient child might have [had] a strong bond with a supportive caregiver, parent, teacher, or other mentor-like figure." Others had a "positive social orientation." "Though not especially gifted, these children used whatever skills they had effectively." [16] Werner also found that "perhaps most importantly, the resilient children had what psychologists call an "internal locus of control": they believed that they, and not their circumstances, affected their achievements. The resilient children saw themselves as the orchestrators of their own fates." [17] Motivation is not magic, it has a lot to do with control, an internal locus of control means we see ourselves as responsible for the quality of our lives, those with an external locus of control have given that control to others or outside of themselves, they react rather than produce.

People with an internal sense of control "were found to perceive less stress, employ more task-centered coping behaviors, and employ fewer emotion-centered coping behaviors than [those with an external sense of control]. Successful internals became more internal, whereas unsuccessful externals became more external over the [the study period]. Changes in performance were related to changes in locus of control." [18] One way to define success is growth; growth-oriented people recognize where choice exists and focus on internal rewards.

Resilience can be learned. We can be less vulnerable, more strong and resilient if we think differently about stimuli, if we "reframe them in positive terms when the initial response is negative"[19] or better regulate emotions says Konnikova. The mental skills needed for resilience can be learned over time permitting us to gain resilience where we previously had none.[20]

Unfortunately, researchers point out that the opposite may also be true. "We can become less resilient, or less likely to be resilient," says psychologist George Bonanno. He adds "We can create or exaggerate stressors very easily in our own minds. That's the danger of the human condition." He adds, "Human beings are capable of worry and rumination: we can take a minor thing, blow it up in our heads, run through it over and over, and drive ourselves crazy until we feel like that minor thing is the biggest thing that ever happened. In a sense, it's a self-fulfilling prophecy. Frame adversity as a challenge, and you become more flexible and able to deal with it, move on, learn from it, and grow. Focus on it, frame it as a threat, and a potentially traumatic event becomes an enduring problem; you become more inflexible, and more likely to be negatively affected," states Bonanno. He adds, "adversity doesn't guarantee that you'll suffer going forward. What matters is whether there is a negative response."[21]

It is easy to live poorly, to be a lousy cop, a mediocre spouse or parent, neighbor or friend, it is hard work to be a good one. The necessary work involves struggle and change. We do best to focus our efforts on what we can control, and manage our reactions to what we cannot control. Sometimes we seek, sometimes we surrender. We persevere towards the internal, not external, ultimately changing ourselves, not the world. We look for our path and stick to it.

CHAPTER 10

PEER SUPPORT AND EARLY INTERVENTION

Help

Know Better

Part of toughness, self-efficacy and even resilience is getting help as needed, but determining when and how can be confusing. Things that we do not understand or are new to us can be mysterious. To give us psychological relief from the tension of the unknown, people might make up wild stories to explain them. Mental health can be very complex and poorly understood. It can be frightening to detect mental and emotional distress or health decline in others.

Seeing others in distress may remind us of our own vulnerability. Sometimes, because of that misunderstanding, our response can be assertively wrong or marked by passivity or avoidance. Whether we do the wrong thing, or do nothing either out of fear or a lack of knowing what to do, in all cases if we know better, we can do better. With education, we can see mental health as less mysterious and officer distress as actually predictable, preventable, treatable, and often ultimately valuable.

If you supervise police officers or intervene when things go wrong, you have a duty to plan ahead. Certain unpleasantries, or in some cases disasters, can be avoided with planning. These unpleasantries include, being surprised, wishing we knew what to do in the midst of it and regretting our action or inaction afterwards. Complex issues like mental and emotional wellbeing do not magically maintain themselves or improve without some effort and forethought, planning and education.

As we have seen on the street, for every crisis there is a "before" the crisis, and there will be an "after" the crisis. We should recognize this same thing happens with a coworker's crisis. Because of convenience, laziness or lack of imagination, we often treat bad things as if they just fell out of the sky. In reality, many bad things are predictable and preventable.

Empathy versus Strategy

When it comes to helping cops, if I were forced to choose between being empathetic or strategic, I would choose the latter. A cop may open up to me because they know I am empathetic, and I hope I am viewed as trustworthy and approachable, but I do not just sit there with a sympathetic look on my face. Actually, sometimes I might, but what I am likely thinking is strategic: "How are we going to get you out of this mess" or "I am glad it has finally come to this and you are ready for a change."

Empathy, the ability to share another person's feelings or "suffer together" in many cases sounds like a bad thing, not automatically a good thing. The Greek Stoic philosopher Epictetus warned against moaning or groaning inwardly.[1] I try to manage my empathic impulses; in fact, I try not to be too empathetic other than to let it alert me to someone's distress. We can be responsive to others, but we need not necessarily suffer as they do. I get a good feeling doing EAP work, but I also have gladly grown suspicious of my own, as well of others' motivation to help. I have come to understand another person's outward signs of distress can make us feel bad. This is especially true for those who pride themselves on their kindness and caring. We may be motivated to decrease their suffering for our own benefit but fail to recognize this. This is why "helping" is not always "helpful." In fact, our "virtuous do-goodery" can cause harm as we may be motivated primarily by our own feelings.[2,3]

I have had only mediocre success communicating this sentiment. It could be because I am wrong about it; however, I do not think so. I am quite sure some people could benefit from becoming more empathetic, but because we hold empathy as so virtuous, we fail to recognize that some empathetic people could benefit from becoming less empathetic. This was true for me. Less empathy and more strategy should not be interpreted as, "I don't give a shit," but more of a rational coolness, a slight detachment, an eager interest in problem solving and identifying a plan to recover and advance wellbeing. I would prefer to think of helping others more as *compassionately strategic*.

A more honest answer to why we want to help others might be if we can reduce their suffering, we can reduce our own. Because we also do not want to cause them harm in pursuit of our own relief, we should hope for some insight as to whether it is best to interject ourselves or to leave people alone. I would rather my actions be guided by necessity and compassion, rather than sympathy. This makes the focus more about their strengths and less about my need to feel better. As do-gooders, we should remain suspicious of our motives. When tempted to offer advice, take some action or create some program, we should consider whether or not we are trying to meet a need of someone in distress or create a need to perpetuate our existence. Understanding this distinction is important because it helps us avoid mental and emotional fatigue and allows us to stay objective about a situation, especially one involving another cop in distress.

Peer Support

Peer support is people using their own experiences to help each other. A peer support team member is a cover officer of sorts whose existence can improve a workgroup's emotional health, wellbeing and sense of belonging. In law enforcement, it allows coworkers to support one another outside of the formal management structure and can be a therapeutic force multiplier and a form of early intervention.

Unlike most careers, in policing we are fortunate to value our tribal ways, depending on our loyalty to each other and a common cause. We survive by interdependence, as we must watch out for each other. It becomes so instinctual that we may not always be aware of it. A cop notices the slightest tone of urgency or stress in another cop's voice on the radio. Two cops, who may barely know each other, or maybe even dislike each other, will walk shoulder to shoulder down a dark alley looking for trouble, positioned to shield and defend the other. There is an "expectation that members will self-sacrifice to contribute to in-group welfare."[4] When a cop calls for help, we will stop at nothing to get to them. And on the receiving end, there is no greater feeling than the sight of them arriving.

There is a part of growth and healing, recovery from harm, that is individual and personal, and there is a part that is communal. Self-awareness and group identity come from both. Experience makes us not better than others, but better for others. As a group, we are *not* as strong as our weakest link, we are as strong as whoever is paying attention, on guard to alert others.

The influence of the group has a powerful impact on each members' behavior and sense of wellbeing. Throughout history, humans' capacity for cooperation and sharing helped us evolve to survive in extremely harsh environments. Our evolution depended on personal interest being subsumed into group interest because personal survival is not possible without group survival. There are obvious psychological stresses on a person in a group, but there may be even greater stresses on a person in isolation. Most higher primates, including humans, are intensely social, and there are few examples of individuals surviving outside of a group.[5]

Maybe the critics of the Thin Blue Line, the police brotherhood-sisterhood, are just jealous, or at the very least ignorant. We need each other and are interdependent in policing in ways the public will never understand, thus it scares them and they criticize it; they insert sinister intent where they could instead be curious. The result can be further police officer estrangement from society.

Our tribal ways are central not only to our street survival, but to our recovery from the cost of doing work that not all of society is able or willing to do. Sebastian Junger argues that conditions like PTSD should be described as a "disorder of recovery" in order to not further alienate and pathologize those that suffer. In this model, the focus is placed on family, community and collective healing.[6]

Keeping this in mind, the means for accessing mental health resources and peer support should maintain some deliberate distance from the administration, including going so far as to shun its embrace. An administration that not only understands this, but actively supports this, will have greater success. A coworkers' mental and emotional problems can be very intimidating, and we might too readily yield control to administrators, therapists or other professionals. But in doing this, we should consider what we lose, services that are peer driven, and arise from those who are closest to the cause and effect can be best. This is not completely dissimilar to when factory line workers are given the authority to improve a product or fix problems that appear before them. Supplied with a set of guiding principles, tools, resources and the authority to use them, groups can fix their own problems.

Peer support, informal or formal, is an important element of wellbeing for police officers. There is no substitution for the understanding, comfort and assistance one cop can give another, only a cop can be a cop to another cop. Add some training and guidance, boundaries and resources and this cop now becomes a healer.[7,8]

What Peer Support Is and Is Not

Peer support means one coworker supporting another. In law enforcement, we can formalize this relationship by creating peer support teams. A peer support team member is a specially selected and trained coworker who distinguishes himself or herself by essentially publicly saying, "I want to help my coworkers with mental and emotional distress." Peer support can provide what fundamentally a cop in distress needs most, which is:

- Someone they recognize and trust,

- Someone they do not need to explain policing to, and

- Someone whose core message is, "Brother/Sister, you are not alone."

Many cops do not need or want therapy, but they may need help seeing things differently. We might call this mentoring, coaching or just being a friend. Relief can come from just expressing their distress to someone else or by way of some kind of feedback.

Peer training includes such topics as confidentiality, respecting boundaries, identifying resources, and probably most importantly, what the role is and what the role is not. For every *to-do* list their needs to be a *do-not-do* list. The goal is to get as clear as possible about the purpose and function of peer support. As a group exercise, during peer training, participants can devise their own lists of what peer support "IS and IS NOT." Below is an example of some responses:

Peer support IS:

Trustworthy
A cop
Familiar, known to them
Good listener
Supportive
Encouraging (provide hope)
Referral to resources as needed
Followup (ongoing connection and checking back)
Helpful
Compassionate
Monitor health of agency
Respect boundaries
Assist EAP
Provide education (with caution)
Advice (with caution)
Voluntary
Help normalize
Protective
Respectful
Early intervention
Permission to feel bad
Uses experience to help others

Peer support IS NOT:

Judgmental
Therapy
About me
Critical
Gossip
Fixer
Advice (with caution)
Identifier of "problem people"
Working for agency, administration, union
Substitute for critical care
Threatening
Psychological evaluation or diagnosis
The Sunshine Club (those at work who might be responsible for organizing gifts, cards, and well wishes for special occasions or events)

Knowing what peer support is not, keeps us focused on what peer support is. Everything cannot be a priority, and if any of us try to be everything to everyone, we will fail. If peer support loses its focus or unity of purpose, it will fail. Peer support team members must agree on what peer support is and is not. The job of the peer support team coordinator is to hold members accountable to what they decide.

A note about giving advice: Advice appears in both lists of what peer support IS and IS NOT. Advice can be presumptuous, unwanted, in some cases inappropriate, harmful and the opposite of good listening. We must examine our motivations, which might be our own discomfort with someone's distress or judgment about their situation. However, advice may have a role, especially because we are not therapists and in a good sense, amateurs. As a guide, we should ask permission before we give advice. Good counsel and guidance may be welcomed, and in some cases underutilized. Sometimes the best we can hope for, as a peer support team member, is to help someone feel a little better or a little less bad. Giving advice, if done honestly and with a sense of compassion and care, can be a brave act that maybe only one cop can do for another.

Why Do It?

Clearly understanding what constitutes help and helping requires some self-examination. This includes the critical realization that "help" is not always helpful, and that the do-gooder can cause serious harm. If the helper is not clear-headed, strong and experienced themselves, they can be part of the problem. Whether you are a member of a peer support team, the EAP director, or designing an EAP system, it is important to remember to not get carried away with our own good intentions.

Each individual must contemplate why they wish to be a peer support team member. The following four questions can be useful in helping sort this out. The first two questions can be part of the application and selection process for prospective team members, and all four questions can be useful as a small group training exercise and large group discussion.

1. Why do I want to be a member of the peer support team?

2. What in my past makes this personally important to me?

3. How is "helping" not always helpful?

4. How can "helping" be truly helpful?

Confidentiality Agreement

A signed confidentiality agreement is like a contract, but more important than any external controls, are internal controls or self-monitoring. A peer support team member will be imperfect of course, but one who talks shit about another cop has forgotten who they are and what they represent. They have become untrustworthy because anyone listening can say, "If this is how they talk about others, this is how they might talk about me." Gossip is inappropriate for peer support team members. Temptations to gossip are an opportunity to demonstrate your trustworthiness by not saying a word or rising above. The manliest thing I ever witnessed a cop do was to halt gossip.

Listening skills

Good listening is a skill and many people may not feel particularly good at it. However, with any skill, you can improve with practice and experience. Some find it helpful to think of good listening as a generosity of time. As you become more comfortable with the discomfort of others, and do not feel the pressure to "fix" them, increasingly you may feel calm in the presence of sadness, anger, or even a crying cop. This makes room for curiosity and a genuine desire to understand what they are feeling.

Listening exercises can be painfully artificial. And if listening becomes a technique, cops will become suspicious that you are using a technique on them. One exercise I have found useful is to divide the group into pairs who have strong opposing views on an uncontroversial topic (NASCAR, hunting, daylight savings time, energy drinks, etc.) and take turns acting as the listener with the following instructions:

- Do not try to educate, try to learn
- Be curious and ask questions to understand why they think and feel the way they do
- Thank them for sharing their views.

The task at hand may often be to just listen, but more likely it is to have a conversation. Think of it as an interview where you are trying to gain the most understanding. And if you do not have time or energy for the conversation, let that be known respectfully.

Celeste Headlee, the author of *We Need to Talk,* reminds us "a conversation requires a balance between talking and listening." Below are a few of her ways to have a better conversation:[9]

- Don't multitask - focus only on the conversation.
- Use open-ended questions.
- Only talk about what you know.
- Don't equate your experience with theirs.
- Listen to truly understand them.

Many of us can recall times when we regret not hearing someone, when in retrospect the other person said what we needed to hear. Sometimes we did not know how to respond, so we pretended not to hear it, or we just plain misinterpreted what was said.

To avoid such lapses, therapists and counselors use a conversation method called motivational interviewing that may be useful in peer support. Fundamentally, this is a conversation style of interacting aimed at strengthening a person's own motivation and commitment to change. Helpful strategies include open-ended questions, affirmations, reflective listening and summarizing what was heard, while avoiding anything judgmental, forceful or giving advice.

A key to good listening is discerning either what people are really saying or the real question underneath the question they are asking. In an anthology compiled by Robert Bly, James Hillman and Michael Meade, there is a poem by William Stafford that describes the hidden meaning in a child's question. In the poem *With Kit, Age 7, At the Beach,* a father and daughter are staring out at a stormy ocean, when the child asks her daddy how far he could swin.[10]

Had the father not recognized the true question, which was the child wanted to be reassured if she was out there in the stormy sea that he could save her, he may have mistakenly answered, "I wouldn't put my toe in that water." But as Michael Mead points out, the child "needs to hear an emotional truth spoken, needs to hear the shape of the father's heart."[11] Wisely the father answered that he could swim as far as needed, and they both understood that in the act of talking, he was swimming out to her. The father reassured his child with the truth, that he would do anything to help her in the "great storms of life."[12]

With practice, my listening skills have improved. I notice I interrupt less and kind of settle into a sort of listening mood when people talk. On some occasions, I feel as if I am sort of half listening, but suddenly I hear something that stands out and I am inspired to take notice or ask a question. With a little more thought and some practice, you will likely have similar results.

Roles for Peer Support Members

The peer support team member activities involve both intake and outreach. Examples of intake are being accessible to coworkers who ask questions about help, support or resources. Outreach involves peer support team members initiating contact with distressed coworkers. The peer approaches a coworker about observed or communicated concerns. The peer is also on the lookout for signs of distress in a specific area of assignment (for example, a particular shift or precinct). During critical incidents or traumatic events, peer support team members can be called upon to assist with post-event Critical Incident Stress Management (CISM) activities and ongoing support. Other contact can include assisting with roll call visits, education, and events that overwhelm the agency.

Because of their personality, experience or reputation, some officers, whether a peer support team member or not, may find that other cops tend to confide in them. This is likely because they are viewed as trustworthy, approachable and maybe empathetic. Other cops are particularly skilled at noticing coworker distress and are able to inoffensively approach them. As peer support team members, they should not rely exclusively on being approached, but must be willing to approach others when concerns seem warranted; otherwise their skills will rarely be used. Approaching others can be intimidating, but the discomfort can lessen and the effectiveness improve with practice and an attitude of genuine concern. You may not know where your actions fit on the spectrum of helping someone else, from bringing the first awareness, to some necessary middle step, to the final transformation. I have had peer support team members later describe these interactions as one of the most rewarding of their careers.

Peer support can be met by a variety of people in a variety of ways, both via responsiveness to intake and courageous outreach. If they are trustworthy, they have a duty to approach someone they suspect is in distress, and likely have all the necessary skills to have an authentic talk with another officer.

Traumatic Event Peer Support Team Outreach

Peer support team members can play an important role in coming to the aid of officers following potentially traumatic events. Just being a member of the team gives them "permission" to start conversations about the mental and emotional impact of "bad calls."

At my agency, when I, or a peer support team member, become aware of a potential traumatic event, we may contact the officer or officers involved. It is simply a personal contact, usually a phone call to check-in with them. I know that if I make more than three or four calls myself I start to sound like a robot, so when the number of potentially impacted officers is large, we share the task among several of us. The phone call is simply a check-in and an acknowledgement of the potentially harmful event. There is no assumption of harm. There are three outcomes when placing the call:

1. You speak with the officer;

2. You leave a message, and they do not call you back;

3. You leave a message, and they call you back.

All three are fine. Officers seem to appreciate most the fact that someone noticed. I have included a guide I created for peer support team members when making these outreach phone calls. Making these phone calls can be intimidating initially. This guide provides instructions and talking points (see pages 191–2).

Why Peer Support Is Good

Police officers are encouraged to have and maintain friendships with those outside of police work, and this is good advice. There is a good reason cops are drawn to each other. We think alike, we act alike, and we trust our shared experience. When officers have mental and emotional struggles, it can be enormously helpful to confide in someone who understands the work and will not judge you for talking disparagingly about the administration and criminals in the same sentence and liberally use the F-word to emphasize your point. Thus, the best resource for a cop before, during and after psychological trauma or mental or emotional distress can be another cop.

PEER TRAUMATIC EVENT OUTREACH
Guide for Peer Support Team When Contacting Officers Involved in a Potentially Traumatic Event

Critical Incidents & Traumatic Events are work-related events that have the potential to temporarily overwhelm coping mechanisms. *Critical Incidents* are defined in policy. The designation of which officers have been involved in a Critical Incident are made at the command staff level and result in a number of mandated EAP interactions. **Traumatic Events are not defined in policy and can best be described as "bad calls," There are no mandated EAP interactions, and when identified, they are handled on a case-by-case basis.**

It is the goal of EAP and the Peer Support Team to be more responsive to and supportive of officers involved in Potentially Traumatic Events. We will accomplish this in part by regularly deploying Peer Support Team members to contact officers involved in Traumatic Events.

How-to Guide and Steps

When: Peer receives a request from EAP Director or Peer Support Team Coordinator. The request for peer assistance will likely be made via text message. Only those peers able and willing need reply.

Who: Officer(s) as assigned. You will be provided with a short list of officer(s) to contact. Ideally, you will also get their tour and cell number.

What: **Steps:**

1. Call/contact assigned officer(s). Make note of possible sleep schedule conflict.
2. Three likely outcomes:
   a.) The officer answers and you talk.
   b.) You leave a message, and they do not call you back.
   c.) You leave a message, and they call you back and you talk.
3. Follow-up later as needed or desired.

Outcomes a, b, or c are all good. You will get better at this type of outreach with experience.

Conversation Tips:

1. Tell them why you called—that you are a Peer Support Team member and you understand they were at this or that event.

2. You are just checking in with them (no one necessarily voiced concerned about them specifically).

3. Ask if it is an okay time to talk briefly.

4. Do Not Assume:

   a.) Everyone you call will have been very involved or negatively impacted.

   b.) They have been harmed in any way, or cannot handle a bad call, or need to see a therapist.

   c.) That feeling bad or having a strong reaction is concerning. It can be a good thing to feel bad about a bad thing.

5. It is useful to ask how involved they were. If they were very involved or appear impacted, a useful conversation starter can be to ask them, *"What was the worst part of it for you?"*

6. Listen, encourage, and refer as needed.

7. If they are concerned about themselves or a family member (i.e., surprised by a strong or lingering reaction, new sleep disturbance, mood change, or feeling stuck) they can contact the EAP director.

8. I end by thanking them for doing the work.

Note: An officer's response to potential psychological trauma remains very individualized. This is due in part to the varied nature of both the event and the officer.

If the officer you speak with expresses concern about another officer, you can contact the EAP director or Peer Support Team Coordinator to see if that officer is on the call list. Additionally, you can encourage the concerned officer to reach out to them as well.

And the best way for an agency to support an officer in distress is to support the supporter.

Access to vetted mental health professionals is necessary when developing systematic approaches to responding to officers who ask for help or are forced to get help. Any system will be an imperfect system, and there will always be important things the experts miss or misinterpret. As an example, our contracted therapists can do ride-alongs or more commonly I will bring him or her out myself. One time, a therapist was riding with me when we arrived on scene as a group of cops managed an angry drunk. The lead cop was nice and kind and said all the right things while another cop lost his patience with the drunk's antics and for lack of a better description, acted a bit unprofessionally.

It was clear to me that the therapist viewed the "nice cop" and the "not so nice cop" as different to the extreme. I explained to her that the angry cop simply got his buttons pushed and to assume that he was maladjusted, and the other not, or that one cop cared deeply for the downtrodden and the other did not, could not be discerned from that demonstration. What was impressive, I told her was how a fellow cop recognized the situation and stepped in inoffensively, as only another cop can, to cool the angry cop down, how cops can watch out for each other and try to keep each other out of trouble.

Cops have robust emotional intelligence that they use on the street to survive and it can be turned inward to support each other. Peers may be best at seeing early signs of trouble in another cop. What cops will always need, and must not be undervalued, is the role of peer support, the work of well-intended and thoughtful non-experts. We cannot do without the insights and sensibilities of these so-called amateurs. Within limits and appropriate caution, we should not defer too quickly to experts or professionals outside of police work.

Many problems are best managed at the lowest level by those closest to the action and do not require therapeutic help. Peer support is well suited for that as long as the peers know when they are over their head or out of their lane. Every peer support team member must have someone they can call and say, "I think I am over my head on this one." This could be the EAP director or a contracted therapist.

Employee Assistance Program (EAP) Services

An Employee Assistance Program is an employer-based program designed to identify and assist employees in resolving behavioral health problems that may adversely affect the employee's performance. These same services can and are provided by organized resources that go by other names such as Officer Wellness, Officer Health and Wellness, but for simplicity, I will continue to use the term EAP.

When trying to navigate the healthcare industry for either physical or mental ailments, it is good to know the language. If we divide health and wellness into physical health and mental health, the term behavioral health is applied to the areas of mental health and addiction. Knowing health care language and processes, especially regarding behavioral health services, is among the responsibilities of EAP staff members.

Most law enforcement agencies provide some kind of EAP. Some are within an organization, while others are independent or contracted to provide serves to the organization. These services can be limited to a list of approved providers to call, or an enhanced EAP where vetted therapists are fully engaged with officers and practices of the agency.

EAP Scalable Design

The principles and basic services of an EAP can be applied to a big or small police department, one with or without an internal EAP. The New York City Police Department has around 40,000 officers. The New York Mills (Minnesota) Police Department has three full-time officers. Both can provide EAP services to its officers.

A successful informal EAP-like system could be an inspired chief, a single dedicated individual within an agency who promotes mental health and wellbeing, or a police culture that maintains high expectations and support for good health and wellbeing. Health insurance plans or even local mental health providers can be asked to do more by way of education and support.

Many law enforcement agencies throughout the United States are small. For these, the best they might expect is a peer support "team" of one, a wellness committee of two. Regionally, smaller agencies can combine efforts and build consortiums to share in support, training, and resources. Certainly, big agencies have big resources, but this is not always an advantage; they can also have overwhelming needs or great difficulty with effective communication and multiple layers of decision making.

With whatever you have, big or small, focus your efforts. Informal peer support likely already exists at any agency, and the goal might be to enhance the skills and access to resources. A wellness committee might already exist in the form of a couple of interested people talking about what could be. For wellness committees or workgroups, they can focus their energies and improve success by defining the committee's purpose and function by answering these questions: How can we support each other's ideas and initiatives? How will we manage and prioritize new or incoming ideas? What "product" will we produce, such as education and outreach?

EAP Services

At my agency, EAP services are available to all department employees, sworn or civilian, and their household family members. Services are provided by the EAP director, peer support team members, and a number of therapists in private practice. I have vetted the therapists and taken them under contract which allows me to set up expectations and an agreed upon reimbursement rate. This is all in addition to the behavioral health resources provided by our health insurance plan.

Specific EAP services vary among agencies. These are the services provided through my agency's EAP:

- Private coaching from EAP director

- Confidential therapeutic sessions from vetted licensed therapists

- Critical Incident response

- Referral to other resources

- Health education

- 24-hour access to EAP contact.

Two functions are fundamental to promoting mental health and wellbeing among police officers: 1) intake and 2) outreach. **Intake** has to do with being accessible and responsive to requests with confidentiality and efficiency. **Outreach** has to do with prevention and health education, trying to get ahead of some of these problems and building protective factors, as well as being on alert to signs of trouble.

The EAP director, peer support team members, trusted coworkers or supervisors can provide private coaching. Qualified and vetted therapists can provide counseling or therapeutic sessions. Regional CISM teams, or specially trained peer support team members and therapists can facilitate critical incident response. Although EAP may be viewed primarily as the route to therapeutic sessions serving a select few, all workers benefit from the education components as well as an elevated expectation of wellbeing. An effective EAP, or EAP-like resources, can set the right tone — that the mental and emotional burden carried by some can be lightened and some specific problems can be "fixed."

Confidentiality. I never try to talk cops out of this very reasonable concern and have never asked a police officer to *trust me*; instead I demonstrate trustworthiness in word and action. I carefully employ a system designed to maintain confidentiality, including such things as a secret contact code to protect the names of officers seeking help. Some cops remain deeply distrustful of the agency and EAP; some would just prefer for a variety of reasons to seek psychological help independent of the police department. This is understandable and there are advantages and disadvantages to both. What is most important is that they get help.

Utilization. While 100% utilization is not the goal, and not all employees need EAP services. All employees need to have confidence in EAP services. High utilization can be viewed as a good thing, not necessarily an indication of increased distress, but instead increased attention to mental health and wellness.

For all industries, the national average EAP utilization is 3-6%.[13] We can imagine that for police officers, the utilization may be even lower. At my agency, some officers are mandated to contact EAP, including officers determined to have been involved in critical incidents, or those under a rare supervisor mandate. The vast majority of officer contact with our EAP is voluntary, or in other words, self-initiated. For comparison, my agency had a 18% voluntary utilization rate for 2017.

If an agency's goal is to maintain productivity and wellbeing, it is unclear if EAPs are effective in this role. If the goal is to provide the employer an option when dealing with troubled employees, that goal is met with the existence of an EAP. Judging outcomes can be difficult, what is within our power is to build useful processes. The level of effectiveness depends on the agency support of the EAP, how well the EAP functions and cops willingness to use it.

Work It

Most important to the success of police EAP is having the right person or persons involved, true believers, a devotee to the cause, who is considered trustworthy and approachable. Continuously, in the forefront of their brain must be three things: maintain confidentiality, represent EAP well, and fiercely protect its reputation.

I make it a priority to see and be seen, cops sometimes tease me that I am trying to get in their heads. If that means being a frequent reminder that EAP services are available and normalizing seeing people talk with me, then yes. My primary motivation is that I am trying to get *them* into *my* head, as I want to understand what they care about, what is going on, what help they may need.

One of the EAP "products" is confidence: providing confidence that EAP will be there for the officer, their family or their partners if needed. The EAP functions best when the cops treat it like their own, a resource they feel safe asking for. EAP is a team approach, where everyone has a role in supporting each other's wellbeing, that includes protecting the reputation of the EAP. I am eager to tell officers that it matters how they talk about EAP. If they do not trust it and have evidence to support a dim view of EAP, then they have a duty to warn other officers. But if they do not, then shut the hell up, because loose talk might dissuade someone from getting the help they need. False claims about EAP may say more about those disparaging it wanting an excuse to avoid asking for help and doing the hard work of getting better.

Do More versus Do Less

New is not always improved, and more is not always better. The struggle to maintain a balance between doing too much and not doing enough is a worthy struggle. The first priorities of managing EAP services are being accessible and maintaining trust. Also important is finding a balance between doing enough but not too much. Like a cop on patrol, every time he interacts with someone, be it a good citizen or a criminal, the officer impacts the next encounter that good citizen or criminal has with the next cop that comes along. With EAP services, it is supremely important that individual officers feel well served.

As an example of how to balance efforts, consider responses to critical incidents. As stated in chapter 5, about two-thirds of officers involved in a critical incident or traumatic events feel bad, or not, for a while and then are ready to go to the next call. About a third are negatively impacted. Most of those officers get better on their own with time, while some get stuck and need additional help. Neither group is necessarily maladaptive. To treat all those involved in critical incident and potential traumatic events as if they were negatively impacted is unnecessary, annoying, and potentially harmful. It may dilute the process of help for those who need it.

Humans are strong and resilient, and most often we manage bad things just fine. Those who are struggling, for whatever reason, have a responsibility to seek help. Because there is no sure way to identify all harmful events, it is better to put the responsibility on those harmed, as well as maintain a team approach where coworkers stay involved in helping each other. After all, there is no central record management system for officer distress. Individuals in distress and those closest to them may be best equipped to take notice and offer help.

I want to build on officers' inherent strengths, not weaken them. The answer to all mental and emotional distress is not therapy; some officers just want or need to talk to someone they trust and who they do not have to explain police work to. My agency was established in 1854 and for the vast majority of that time there has been no EAP or established therapeutic resources. Cops have watched out for each other, sometimes very effectively, both with and without an EAP. We do not want to replace that, but instead add to it. At the same time, friends, coworkers and coaches have to be alert to the limits of their role or ability to help in some cases when a cop wants or needs professional help.

It is hard to make things better and easy to make things worse. One nagging concern I have as our EAP becomes more known and effective is that it will inadvertently replace, undermine, or damage the long-standing organic systems of watching out for each other. I do not want cops thinking the EAP director or a peer support team member will parachute in to offer support to a distressed cop while they are standing right next to them and do not help.

The role of the EAP is not to be in charge of all problems, or hover over cops looking for signs of distress, but to connect the need with the help, and make that process as palatable as possible. Striving to maintain a balance between too much and too little means there are times I risk underachieving while I avoid overstepping or being overly eager to help. Ideally, people get mostly what they need and the process does not cause harm. A valid outcome is having participants have a good experience after which they become advocates of EAP services.

Because resources are limited, it is best to focus mental health efforts on education and access to voluntary assessment and trusted resources. Some have advocated for an annual mental health check for officers. This *seems* like a good idea, but agencies must consider the financial costs and unintended consequences. Unless an agency is fully prepared to effectively deal with what they find, there is a real hazard in unscrewing the top of someone's head so to speak, poke around inside, and when what is found frightens us, try to get the lid back on again. A psychological assessment of any workgroup will reveal a percentage of people with sometimes alarming mental and emotional distress. It is unethical to start something like this if you are unprepared to finish what you start. Additionally, some people need their coping mechanisms, even so-called dysfunctional ones, intact and unmolested, to survive their work day the best they know how, as is their right.

I have visited EAPs at other agencies, and I know that there are a variety of ways to provide these fundamental services and more. I am confident there are some gems out there that I do not know about, that are innovative, effective and well-received.

Blue Light Example

If we look across the ocean to the United Kingdom we find an impressive organization called Blue Light Programme (www.mind.org.uk/bluelight), which provides mental health support for emergency services staff and volunteers from ambulance, fire, police and search and rescue services across England and Wales.[14]

Blue Light is a comprehensive region-wide approach and, among many other contributions, it has made peer support a priority. The program offers numerous resources and practical ideas for peer support programs. I have found the Blue Light program to be one of the best sources for innovative and practical ideas to support the mental health and wellbeing of public safety personnel.

Early Intervention

Early interventions are deliberate actions to both prepare for and respond to distress, but more importantly, try to prevent harm in the first place. The goal is to reduce the harms associated with known problems, reduce risk behaviors and develop protective factors. These actions include pre-event education, assessments and specific treatments targeted at common problems or ailments. All of these actions have the potential to be both preventative beforehand or reduce harm afterwards.

Early intervention is *anti-crisis*, trying to get ahead of some problems, simply acting sooner rather than later. Operating on the assumption that by the time most cops ask for help or get forced to get help, a lot of unnecessary damage has been done, and in some cases too much damage to save jobs, marriages, or health. Generally, the longer a problem goes without treatment, the harder it is to treat, and "hitting bottom," as in the case of alcohol addiction or other mental health problems, may mean death, not skid row. The intent is that in areas such as psychological trauma, general mental and emotional distress, and substance use, we can in effect bring the bottom up by preparing all cops with pre-event education, nudging them towards assessment and treatment as needed, and use the benefits of our tribal ways to support recovery and on-going health and wellbeing.

Some early intervention efforts can be specific to an event, issue or symptom such as prolonged sleep disturbances, relationship conflicts, or drinking problems. Some problems can be identified as a specific symptom related to a specific event, but more often it seems they are a generalized decline unrelated or not necessarily traceable to a specific event. Additionally, agencies must do what they can to reduce general work frustration. Specific events or not, early intervention is intended to act early, not late.

Education

In patrol work, when responding to a call for service we often do just the minimum to make the problem go away, clear up the call and go to the next one. We are not in charge of all of society's dysfunction, and trying to get to the core of each issue may not be our job. Sometimes the problem solves itself; sometimes it gets a lot worse. But in some cases, if we do not fix or alter the core issue we will get called back again.

With officer distress, we may need to go beyond just responding, guided by the recognition that all mental and emotional distress has a before, during and after. In other words, the during is an officer's angry outburst that generates a complaint, or the after is his arrest for drunk driving, or the taking of his own life. Reacting effectively, as well as intervening early, require an understanding of a before, during and after, with more emphasis on the before.

The before is all the buildup, all the preceding events. From an educational point of view, this is an opportunity to learn about risk factors, strengthen prevention factors and support behavior changes. While reacting is a focus on getting through an event, early intervention is a focus on prevention, minimizing harm, normalizing and speeding recovery to keep people whole.

Education is an essential element of early intervention; however, education is often treated as an afterthought, as something nice to do, not a thing we must do and must do well. This will likely continue, in part because of our nature, our cop-like impatience and desire to get to the action; we skip over education and just start doing, even if it is half-assed or wrong. And when we do act, often that means we were taught the minimum from someone that knew the minimum, and over time the quality of doing the task or correctly attending to a problem degrades. So, it is important to know about the challenges of quality education.

Preparation and instruction to address mental and emotional problems include forming questions, considering what-if scenarios, consulting experts, and studying the issues and solutions. In short, identifying what to avoid and what to seek. Education intends to persuade the audience to claim the goals for themselves and realize lasting behavior change. The benefits of effective education may never be fully known because bad outcomes can be prevented.

Training Example

Consider officer seatbelt use as an example of a training or behavior change. An individual officer may commit to wearing her seatbelt because her daughter asked her to, another officer because he saw the deadly results of an officer not wearing one. But what about a group of officers?

When I was a patrol supervisor I wanted more of my cops to wear seatbelts more of the time. I felt this was a realistic goal, and I intended to be effective in my efforts. So rather than yell at them in roll call about how it is the policy, I devised a plan that over time would allow me to reach all the cops. Each tour, at the end of roll call I would matter-of-factly read a small list of cops' names and tell them I wanted to speak with them as a group in my office. I did not soften the anxiety of letting them think they were in trouble. When the group assembled I started by telling them my mission statement, I remained standing, looked them in the eyes and said, "I want each of you to wear your seat belts more often." I proceeded with the following steps:

1. I read them the policy, which essentially states they must follow state law.

2. I then read the state statute, which I would point out had an exception allowing for certain non-wearing situations that could be applied to police work. Knowing there are exceptions and an all-or-none approach would fail, I told them I did not want them wearing their seat belt all the time, like when cruising an alley for example. (Fresh in our minds was a recent line-of-duty death where the ambushed officer killed was found wearing his seatbelt.)

3. I then told an ambulance story, illustrating when you roll your squad for example, it is all about physics and your body will find its way out of any opening in the car and you will rag-doll fly through the air. "You owe it to your family and the rest of us to not die that way," I cautioned them.

4. Next, I told them I wanted a 25% increase in seatbelt use starting today. (The 25% was a random number, intended to get the non-wearers started and the sometimes wearers to increase, effecting a whole-group effort and improvement.)

5. Next, I looked each of them in the eye and asked each officer to make a spoken commitment and shake on it.

6. Lastly, I offered them seatbelt extenders that I got for free from Ford.

Later, two young cops sent me photos that showed them wearing their seatbelts. A pair of older cops, who had previously been committed non-seatbelts users, said they thought they could do 25% and said the handshake put them over.

Assess and Treat

Assess and treat involves recognizing the signs and symptoms of certain mental health problems. In some cases, rather than waiting for problems to become known or result in significant harm, I try to nudge them towards a proactive response, in effect trying to find early signs of trouble. Every year I pick two wellness issues I will focus on for the year. My approach is to introduce the subjects, provide routes to confidential self-assessments, and offer access to appropriate therapeutic or treatment resources for those who request it. Complying with recommendations is voluntary. Topics that work well with this approach are alcohol misuse, psychological trauma, sleep problems and healthy relationships.

―――――――

Some cops naturally gravitate toward formal or informal peer support roles, or find themselves frequently coaching junior officers or those they supervise. Our number one unique qualification is that we are another cop. Add to this, trustworthiness, some training, and knowledge of resources, and we become a wellness force multiplier.

PART III

LIVE WELL

PEOPLE-DOORS-HIDES. BEING COPS, WE SEE HOW PEOPLE really live. We witness both their good and bad behavior; we see them when they are victimized with their defenses down. No one enters more homes than cops, seeing people as they are, not just as they wish to be seen. We are uniquely positioned to observe and participate in the lives of others, and with some self-reflection, we can use that experience for our own self-improvement and to live more deeply, to value and nurture both our outer and inner life.

If we call this experience a journey, it is a lifelong one that continuously requires that we adapt and grow, both internally, and in regards to our relationships and connection to the community. With clarity about our purpose and function, we can feel like our best self, our truest and natural self, fully engaged in our lives.

I became a cop relatively late in life, and my happiness as a police officer could have been a function of my age, not in spite of it. I have found police work to be good, honest, soulful work. As a patrolman, I regularly had moments of bliss, I could probably garner more favor if I said otherwise, but it would not be true, I loved the work. Any job can be done soulfully, but police work begs for it.

For me to offer advice or commentary on inner life, outer life, and about clarity of purpose to anyone but my own children might be presumptuous. But these are things I have been contemplating for as long as I can remember, and I am convinced they are fundamental to wellbeing. To not include them in a health and wellness book is remiss and makes all other commentary uninspired. I will not try to tell you where you need to go and how you get there, because I do not exactly know where there is; however, you are on a journey and it useful to give thought to your inner and outer life to gain greater clarity of purpose. It is essential to live well. I will not hide my long and enduring belief that this whole journey is a spiritual one, I believe this because it is part of the human experience. If I am wrong, or this is offensive, you can dismiss it as my bias.

CHAPTER 11

INNER AND OUTER LIFE

Save Yourself

Inner Life

I lean towards the spiritual and believe that our best life requires attention to both our inner and outer life. I believe to live well, you must have clarity about your purpose and function. An inner life might be described as the relationship we have with ourselves, the world that seems within; an outer life as the relationship we have with others or the outside world. Where the two meet is our sense of self, connected to each other, with endless depth and possibility. Those relationships need not be thought of as linear, going out in opposite directions. And if they are, this might indicate a critical imbalance, too much of one thing. Instead we might conceive of them as circular. As I explore my inner self, I discover a connection to all things; and as I examine my relationship to the outer world, I discover a power greater than myself or a connection to all things as well. Some of our deepest happiness comes in the act of exploring the unexplored.

Examined Life

Plato, a student of Socrates, wrote, "An unexamined life is not worth living."[1] Self-reflection is not selfish. There are powers and influences in the world that will pull us along, and if we do not pay attention, we can end up somewhere we did not want or intend to be. Giving attention to an inner life is a way to direct your life. Rather than be a passive participant in it, you will counteract the mind-numbing dominate culture, and bring yourself back to the center. Maybe this is why prayer, meditation, or walks in the woods can feel like centering yourself.

In northern Minnesota, there is a region called the Iron Range where you can tour a mineshaft and travel a half-mile underground where iron ore was once excavated. There, the darkness is so pure, it is disorienting, and a quiet so great that you can hear your heart beating. We live in a world with a lot of noise and distraction, much of it coming from within. If we can quiet that noise, even for brief periods, an inner voice can be made known, an ancient wisdom that was always there, but unheard. After going into the mineshaft, whether in a real or figurative way, when we return to the surface, we can be a better partner, spouse, parent, coworker, and citizen. We become better hosts for our own best selves.

Self-Reflection

I have often thought many people hold high ideals, but few have had them tested as police officers do. The ongoing test of one's courage, and the endless exposure to the suffering of others, beseech officers to continuously examine their own life. Police work offers an unusual opportunity for mental and emotional progress through self-examination and facing what is revealed.

What is revealed might come like a flash of clarify, an ah-ha moment, a path suddenly made obvious. Just as likely, self-reflection might be a simple nudge in a different direction, or a diminishing of interest in something that once was appealing and is no longer so. Self-reflection can be messy and hard on the ego. Like when you realize that your criticism of others says more about you than them. For example, a particular trait or annoying behavior of another may get your attention because what they are doing or not doing, is something you wish you could do or not do.

Forgiveness

As a young boy, I learned the fundamentals of forgiveness from school and church, as well as from what my parents said and maybe more importantly did not say about others. My childhood view of forgiveness was that it was related to a sin or festering wrong that needed righting. All of this was usually applied long after the fact and required a request of another or of God. Over time, I expanded my understanding of forgiveness. As a young man, I became aware that people could express their internal pain and suffering in hostile or disagreeable behavior and recognizing this I was able to "forgive" offensive behavior and respond to them with greater latitude. I will not claim success here, just ongoing effort.

It may be helpful to know that inclinations towards compassion occupy different areas of the brain than does fear, so it is difficult or maybe impossible to entertain both at the same time. We might consider that fear can block or obstruct access to love and compassion. Some describe fear and love as the opposite ends of a spectrum, where we are continuously challenged to choose between the two. Self-compassion, receiving compassion, or gifting it to others, can transcend fear. Compassion acts as a major antidote to relieving the effects of the heightened fear state experienced during difficult times.[2]

The fruit of forgiveness includes freedom from the harm that withholding forgiveness causes us. Thus, forgiveness of others can be a gift we give to ourselves. In forgiveness, we are not being asked to disremember, though that may be part of it, but instead, to loosen a grievance's grip on us. One definition of forgiveness is "giving up all hope for a better past."[3] Some believe life progress depends on all of us eventually forgiving both our mother and father for any experienced or perceived shortcomings. In some cases, the gift of forgiveness can be applied in real-time to ourselves when we make mistakes due to misguided self-centeredness, insecurity or fear. I have found an internal mantra of "Do the next right thing" useful when I felt I had made a mistake in thought or action.

We know in police work that fear can be useful, and we need not devalue fear. Sometimes it is fine to not feel any obvious emotions. Cops may have experienced the cool detachment from emotions when confronting danger. We may not want to, or be able to, force love or forgiveness to occupy a space held by fear. Fear usually gets its way and may dominate our thoughts. At the same time, we can be afraid of intense feeling or painful thoughts. This is why therapeutic processes can be useful to help us move on, lessen fear or other strong emotions attached to some painful memories, thus making room for compassion and forgiveness.

Distress

It is important to recognize when something is not right, and a warning device is built into us, registering dis-ease, dis-stress, or dis-comfort. We cannot help but want to move past these feelings, and maybe our greatest fear when we feel distress is that it will last forever. But we must pause to acknowledge it, and in some cases be willing to go deeper into distress. See dis-stress as a friend.

Sometimes distress is a sign of being out of balance. Distress might be alerting us to something missing or underdeveloped, and the pursuit of that may require a focus that verges on obsession for awhile.

Self-Improvement

How best to live? At some point it seems, everyone must stop and examine where they are and compare that to where they hope to be. Unless guided by some principles, we will rely only on our most basic instincts to seek pleasure and avoid pain, which could include remaining distracted or anesthetized. I know no other way to advance our wellbeing then to actively move between seek or surrender. Keep a higher purpose in mind while focusing your attention on the next step. A daily routine of self-reflection can take this form, a process in the morning reflecting on your values through such things as study, prayer, meditation, or journaling. An evening process where you reflect on your successes and failures in regard to your values. It is useful to study any text you may feel inspired to read or use as a guide.

Mindfulness

Mindfulness, in the simplest terms, refers to the experience of living in the present moment. Cops experience this with some frequency on the job, and it is not probably what the yogi had in mind. For example, when the cop is reacting to a dangerous suspect thinking, "Your next move determines mine." There is nothing like a potentially life threating situation to get you to live in the here and now. Living in the moment can feel really good, it makes us feel more alive.

When thinking of the things that make us feel alive, a cop might confuse this mindfulness with an adrenaline rush. Adrenaline rushes certainly make you feel alive, but they are not sustainable and are largely out of your control. Additionally, like a drug, you may need higher and higher "doses" to achieve the same "high." In contrast, mindfulness is within your control.

Mindfulness can be practiced intentionally, by non-judgmentally drawing your attention to the present moment, or arrive naturally as we fully engage in certain activities. In our personal lives, these activities could be laughing or playing games with our friends and family, hunting, traveling, gardening, fishing (thinking about fishing), or maybe even cleaning the garage can be enlivening because of the novelty or meditative quality of a simple routine or singular focus. But few of us can, or even expect to, live in the moment day-to-day, as our lives can be a blur of responsibility and demands, sometimes filled with unnerving uncertainty and ambiguity.

The kind of mindfulness cops need is the kind that quiets the mind, settles the breath, and connects with an inner wisdom. For some people, this might be prayer, an important pause, meditation, or joyful pursuits. Developing mindfulness skills takes practice and increasingly bears fruit over time, or might arrive in a moment of gratefulness. Either way, through effort or non-effort, it can be helpful to think of mindfulness as righting yourself in the moment, like recalibrating or centering something that is out of balance.

Mindfulness can quiet the mind, but it can wake it as well; this means being more conscious or mindful of what are we doing and where we are we going. Once when I fell asleep on a train, a stranger woke me, somehow she knew I was going to miss my stop. Continuing past my stop would not have been the *end of the line* for me, but it would have taken me farther from my destination. As a child, I was awakened to mindfulness through prayer and meditation, it seems only right to alert others of a chance to get off the train they are on.

The subject of mindfulness is as big as the universe, and the more I try to say, the more I may only reveal my ignorance. In an attempt to say less, not more, I venture to comment only on two topics, prayer and meditation. For some people, these are the same, for others, distinctly different. We might think of prayer as involving words, meditation the absence of words. However, they might both meet in the same space, a kind of transcendence.

Prayer

Note: I know that some people may have been harmed by religion and all its duplicity, crimes and the hypocrisies of practitioners and representatives. I am sorry for that, but point out that organized religions do not *own* God or spirituality, and they have no power to separate you from whatever form of prayer can be yours.

Prayer, which can be both an individual or group activity, may be reciting prepared words or a kind of deeply personal ad lib. Prayer implies communication with God or a power greater than yourself.

When my grandmother, a good lifelong Lutheran, expressed doubt to me near the end of her life, I was shocked. Maybe I thought that a lifetime of devotion and service would have built up enough points to secure a sense of confidence when you finally neared the front of the long line. But now when I think of it, she was expressing fear, not knowing what was next. The thought gives me a sense of compassion for myself and others. Life can be hard, and it is scary. Faith can be at the very least comforting, but it is illusive and sometimes that relationship can feel one-sided, which might be the experience of doubt. Faith cannot eliminate darkness. Even Jesus appeared to have his doubts, and he *was* God. Doubt may be a part of faith, not an antithesis or some proof against God. I have been very confident and wrong, other times, felt lost and alone and been comforted by something outside myself. Some might argue that faith in God is a human invention. I suppose that might be true but if so, it was created for a good reason, because the moment we fall asleep we must put our trust in what the universe has created. Certainty about God is probably unavailable, and I can live with that.

I feel I would be hiding something if I discussed the subject of an inner life without acknowledging the role of prayer in my daily life. I have spent a lot of time praying, mostly of the ad lib sort, experiencing both a free and natural flow, and what might be heard as a clumsy and forced one-way conversation. Either way, at the very least, I show up every day. My time in prayer is not a measure of piety, just a statement of fact. I also got an early start. In fact, I don't remember a time that I was not "God conscious." I was prayed for before I was born, and my mother told me that as a baby she held me in front of a picture of Jesus in our house and repeated his name to me. I saw my father kneeling in prayer at his bedside, we attended church as a family and prayed before meals. I remember the moment when it occurred to me that not everyone I knew said a nightly prayer before going to bed. I know people in recovery who daily kneel in prayer, giving thanks for their unlikely survival to a power greater than themselves.

Sometimes prayer has only bordered my day, a morning and nighttime ritual. In other periods in my life, I felt I was in constant prayer (the time I found myself standing literally in wet cement was during the constant prayer period). Or another period that lasted years, when I was in a sort of spiritual desert and my prayer life was sustained only by habit, trying to stay connected. That was a spiritually painful time; it felt like I had been kicked out of a club of two, me and God. I remember distinctly feeling that it was for my own good, that I was maintaining a false and immature view of God, and I had to surrender what I had known to make room for something new. There were other times that prayer felt like a lifeline, at one particularly difficult stretch I repeated a prayer, sometimes several times an hour, to keep me sane.

> Dear God, my desire, my priority is inner peace.
> I want the experience of love.
> I don't know what would bring that to me.
> I leave the results of this situation in your hands.
> I trust your will. May will your will be done. Amen[4]

Possibly the most ecumenical prayer, one that is known by even "nonbelievers" is the Serenity Prayer which is often associated with Alcoholics Anonymous and Twelve-Step recovery.

Noteworthy is that in an article titled, "Our nation's greatest contribution to religious thought is Alcoholics Anonymous," the author points out that "A.A.'s meeting rooms are where postmodern men and women gather regularly, not because they are 'supposed to' but because it is a matter of survival. The miracle they rediscover there is that by telling their own story of brokenness and listening to others' stories they are somehow moved toward healing. It is a communion of people who recognize that in moving beyond themselves and serving others they find greater peace and wholeness. Sounds a lot like church to me."[5]

The Serenity Prayer is actually derived from a quote attributed to the Greek philosopher Epictetus, "Happiness and freedom begin with a clear understanding of one principle: Some things are within your control, and some things are not. It is only after you have faced up to this fundamental rule and learned to distinguish between what you can and can't control that inner tranquility and our effectiveness become possible."[6]

Most people know only the first part of this prayer, but I have included a contemporary version of Reinhold Neiburhr's entire prayer here.

Serenity Prayer
God grant me the serenity
to accept the things I cannot change;
courage to change the things I can;
and wisdom to know the difference.
Living one day at a time;
enjoying one moment at a time;
accepting hardships as the pathway to peace;
taking, as He did, this sinful world
as it is, not as I would have it;
trusting that He will make all things right
if I surrender to His Will;
that I may be reasonably happy in this life
and supremely happy with Him
forever in the next.
Amen[7]

There are ancient prayer practices and rituals that can and do serve people well today, but equally inspiring is what I heard Anne Lamott say while describing her go-to prayers, "Help me, help me, help me" or "Thank you, thank you, thank you." Someone told me that she later added a third prayer, "Wow!"

For me, there are times when my prayers are structured and specific, including combining prayer with the study of sacred text or other inspirational readings, other times just a quick hello. Some prayers were more like an apology, others like a shopping list. After all these years, I can say that I am still not sure how to pray, but I have become increasingly relaxed about the imperfection of it all. Daily, sometimes hourly, I want most to quiet my mind and feel connected to God, to pause and take notice of my life, to express angst and sometimes complain bitterly, but mostly to give thanks. My relationship with God has evolved, or maybe more accurately, my discovery of God continues to change. If God is what I think God is, I am reassured that we do not have to get it exactly right.

Meditation and Breathing

Thinking of meditation as a skill that needs practice can seem odd to a novice. Some people think of meditation as having to practice doing nothing, and that may be true, but doing nothing is harder than one might think. A lot of things compete for our attention, both inside us and out, and it can be very challenging to "do nothing," and it is different than zoning out in front of a TV. It is difficult to quiet the thinking mind.

Meditation takes a variety of forms. It can be a specific practice or discipline, but in its purest form, it is arriving at a mental state of being, which feels centered and free of any distress. Meditation might be sitting in a quiet space seeking a kind of emptiness of thought, guided by what is sometimes described as conscious or mindful breathing, sometimes called breath work. For some, meditation could be a walk in the woods and being restored by nature.

The absence of thought, or enjoying a singular focus, can come naturally during pleasure and play, and the pursuit of what gives us joy. The practice of meditation is purposefully introducing, or maybe more correctly, making a space for just resting in a state of being.

The meditation process or technique involves these basic steps:

1. Get comfortable and softly close your eyes.

2. Observe your breath as it moves through your nostrils, noticing as it goes in, and out.

3. When your mind wanders, bring it back to your breathing.

Your mind will wander. The practice part or skill building occurs when you notice your mind wandering and bring your attention back to your breathing, notice and start over, notice and start over, notice and start over.

It is useful to remove judgment about what distracts you. This can be put into practice by only giving casual notice of thoughts, sounds or sensations. Let them come and go as if they all have equal weight. Have faith that of all the thoughts and concerns you hold in your head, the most important ones will still be there when you return. Imagine yourself before all your thoughts, worries and concerns, without all your aches, pains and troubles. You can end the session with the thought, "I only have this day."

Be patient with yourself, you are breaking a lifetime habit of constant thinking and not focusing on the here and now. You are learning a new skill and it takes repeated cycles of trying and starting again. Just showing up and trying is an accomplishment. If you find it seemingly impossible to not think about other things, and you feel worse, consider repeating a phrase or a sound.

A common struggle for those seeking to meditate are distracting thoughts, such as to-do lists or concerns about time. Anxiety about these thoughts only make it worse. One approach is to simply acknowledge them and then go back to a focus on breathing. Another person described his method, "I imagine that I'm leading a docile mule down a trail, the mule is sometimes distracted by something along the path, I do not beat the mule into submission, I gently guide it back to the path and we continue."

Like prayer, meditation can be a routine to which we dedicate time and space, but just as valid is a moment of pause; you breathe deeply and look in the direction of your center. This can be just as valuable and easier to work into your daily life.

Conscious Breathing. Deliberately focusing on your breathing is a centering or relaxation technique in and of itself. Here are two techniques you can try. The key is a slow exhalation.

Pause what you are doing, get comfortable, notice your breath as it comes in your nose, into your chest and out your nose again. Allow your breathing to be natural and relaxed. Notice the sensation in your nose, chest or belly. If distracted, gently bring your attention back to the sensation of your breathing. If you wish, mentally recite, "in goes the good air, out goes the bad" or any other phrase that works for you.

Square or box breathing is another technique where you breath in for a count of four. Hold your breath for a count of four. Breath out for a count of four. And then hold your breath for a count of four.

Time
Despite all our advances, technology and supposed time-saving gadgets, we seem to live a more hectic life than our ancestors. Less time for prayer,

meditation, calm conversation with neighbors and friends, meals with our family. Even if our ancestors had less "free time," the pace of their work and responsibilities was different. Even driving a car was mostly just driving a car, maybe listening to whole songs on the radio and pleasantly looking out the window. Our life pace may be more of a choice than we like to admit, and so-called multitasking may be a myth that can mean we just do a lot of things poorly.

Mindfulness is a stopping and looking around, pausing to rebalance the mind-body connection, to ask what am I doing and why, or just to relax or connect with an internal or universal wisdom, to experience just being, even briefly, without all the layers of thought and responsibility. Otherwise we might just be getting to the wrong place in a hurry.

Joy

There is a deep good feeling we can learn to recognize that can be our guide. The trick can be differentiating it from the relatively shallow good feeling associated with avoidance of pain or satisfying a craving. The best word might be joy, tranquility or peace: feeling connected to others through laughter, restored by engaging with nature, experiencing gratitude, or meditating on the thought that you lack nothing.

All this talk of an inner life, prayer and serenity need not conflict with being a police officer. In fact, I have found no conflicts between my religious or spiritual life and police work. The only conflict is the age-old struggle between one's ideals and living up to them. Along the way, I wish only to be judged by my actions, and I see no reason we cannot be both fierce and kind.

Outer Life

Some people may primarily think of their life in terms of their outer life, rarely reflecting on their own thoughts or inner life. The outer life might be understood to be an extension of the inner life where we interact with friends, family and the community as a whole. The nature of police work means you are involved in the community at a very real level, and sometimes with a skewed perspective. Since we have addressed our work interactions with colleagues, supervisors, and the community in other chapters, let us focus mostly on our loved ones here.

Our Neglected Loved Ones

Essentials of a valued and committed relationship include honesty, loyalty, communication, respect, and thoughtfulness. At the sad and destructive other extreme of this are abuse and extramarital affairs. Officers have expressed to me surprise by the unfaithfulness of a spouse, seemingly unaware of the officer's neglect and absence in form of physical presence, emotional availability or even abuse that led up to it. Right or wrong, a spouse will seek what he or she needs most — either becoming numb without it or going elsewhere to find it.

The other side of this is when the cop is the one seeking an affair. I have noticed the affair seeking behavior has a parallel to addiction or chasing the high. Thinking the perfect "other" is mostly a fantasy, fueled by the sexual hit or high of the pursuit, they are seduced by a false belief that this new person is the solution and their committed relationship is so broken.

Cops should not wait for relationship troubles to become a crisis, but recognize it can be the result of under-performing, under-enjoying, and under-appreciating their loved ones. If we lack some skills or right frame of mind, it could be because we were never taught or had healthy role models for being a good husband, wife, father or mother. We do not necessarily automatically know how to be these things. Committed relationships are very challenging, they force growth and the necessary skills can be learned.

Our Loved Loved Ones

Our loved ones are those such as a spouse, partner, children, the family or other committed relationships we have. They all are special to us, want to be treated special and should be. The problem is that police work, as well as other occupations, can be so demanding that we routinely use up our best selves at work, and they get what is left over.

So, it takes constant and deliberate efforts to:

1. not work too much;

2. not enjoy too much "cop specialness," letting being a cop take over all aspects of your life; and

3. make daily choices to save some of your best self for your loved ones.

Working Too Much

Imagine a health fair at a police department with booths offering cholesterol checks, free stress balls, massages and so on. Missing would be a booth that promotes working less off-duty/overtime or none at all. I understand the potential financial hardship, but cops need to recognize what they give up in working too much and the risk of working themselves to death. An alternative to needing more money is needing less money, needing less because of choices to keep your cost of living lower. Sometimes the freedom we seek comes from wanting less, not accumulating more.

When working all the time starts to feel normal and being at home strange and foreign, you are in trouble. Kind of like the warning that when you are thirsty, you are already dehydrated. Time away from work is important, but maybe more important is just spending more time at home. Cops occasionally share with me their conversations with therapists, but rarely do they acknowledge what I happen to know is commonly advised — work less.

Cop Specialness. Our work schedule and demands can take over the family schedule. It is like the family becomes the cop's support crew. Not every work week should become a car race with your family acting as your pit crew. There are certain times and situations that you require extra help and support, but it should be the exception not the routine. It is okay to think you are special while at work, but when you get home and walk through the door you better get over your specialness and get over it quick. Your job is no more special than anyone else's job at home.

Daily Choices. Police work can be very seductive, make great demands of time and energy and like a shiny object, distract us from our sometimes-mundane tasks, responsibilities and simple pleasures of home life. It is essential that officers are deliberate in their efforts to find a balance with work and home life. An interesting observation I have made is that some very "average" cops have fabulous personal lives, are devoted to their loved ones and have a lot of joy away from work, while some "super cops" sometimes have what might be considered disastrous personal lives.

A cop must be *useful* at home or risks slowly becoming *useless*. Your family will learn to live without you. It is arguable that doing laundry, cleaning the bathroom, preparing meals and helping the kids with homework not only makes you an engaged family member, but a better cop.

Marriage requires that you look at how your behavior affects another and having children "wrecks" your previous life in a good way. It forces growth because a spouse and children require that you constantly make adjustments, accommodations and compromises for the needs of the whole, not just yourself. A committed relationship, whether to a life partner or a child, forces growth towards whole-heartedness. To be something for someone else, whether as a partner, parent or guardian, we must go beyond or outside of our own needs.

I have been married for over 30 years, but remarkably have very little advice to give, other than to say this: The things you value need time and attention, and more than just keeping them fed and watered, they need to be enjoyed.

Reassure Them

Loved ones (including children) need to be reassured about the dangers officers face when they are ready to hear it. It is likely best to be open and straightforward about some of the risks and not give false promises of guaranteed safety.

It can be very reassuring to our loved ones to know more about your training, what you pay attention to and how you do your job: your ability to be suddenly fierce on demand, the peer pressure to be smart and safe, and how we often move around like a wolf pack, check on each other at traffic stops, keep a mental map of where each other is and listen carefully to the inflection of each other's voice, as well as the oversight from dispatchers and supervisors that monitor our status.

Additionally, loved ones should know that cops often know when they are approaching danger. Loved ones may have the false impression that they are in a danger zone the entire shift, where in fact, while a family might be at home concerned, their cop has his or her boots off typing a boring-ass theft report or laughing and joking with co-workers in the safety of the headquarters.

Suit of Armor (Kevlar)

We wear a badge as a representation of the guardian or warrior's shield. Our skill, experience and mental toughness are our suit of armor. But there is no amount of armor or Kevlar to keep us from harm in all situations. We also need the agility and alertness that comes with being well-fed, well-rested and well-loved. Our loved ones provide this other type of protection, a shield that they place on us, emblazoned with the family crest. These loved ones are whose pictures are on our lockers, whose images have come into the mind of cops in the midst of the fight for their life, whose honor we protect and whom we return home to. That shield is repaired and polished at home and among friends, the place where we remove the suit of armor. That armor and what it protects does not belong only to the cop, but the family and the community.

Cops go through a mental process when putting the armor on, preparing themselves. They should give as much mental energy to taking it off, mentally preparing to return home and be their best for their loved ones. The work-to-home transition can be difficult and requires some deliberate planning and negotiation. One cop described it this way, "My first day off I sleep extra, workout, be kind of selfish, day two and three, I'm expected to be all the way back into family mode." I heard one woman whose father was a cop say, "We all gave him 30 minutes when he got home to take his cop face off."

Work "Family"

I am opposed to referring to a workplace as a family, the *police family* for example. I understand why we do it. We spend time together, and we understand and need each other. Those who use the phrase may have wished to express their gratitude for the kindness shown them after suffering a loss or the closeness they feel sharing good times and bad. Or to acknowledge that they care deeply about their coworkers and are comforted by knowing others care about them. For some, loyal coworkers might be the closest thing they have to a family. In many ways we are *like a family*, including all the dysfunction and intense feelings, and frank expressions of likes and dislikes that many families experience. We rely on each other, risking life, limb and reputation as we move shoulder-to-shoulder towards danger, sometimes with other cops we hardly know, but with whom we share the same patch on our sleeve. In that moment, we are devoted to a common cause, and are interdependent for literal survival. Other cops we know very well, and being trained observers, we can see when troubles at home or work disillusionments are wearing on them. Like a family we love, hate, like, dislike, and tolerate all kinds of quirks and idiosyncrasies of people we are stuck with.

However, a workplace is an organization or institution, it is incapable of caring about you — only individual people can do that. The workplace is not a family, it is a workplace, and we can feel love and devotion towards coworkers without calling them family.

Police work is dangerous, to the family as well. Here is the danger, if we use the word *family* to refer to our work friends and acquaintances, what does it say about our family at home? What does it say to the home family if a cop literally has an affair with a member of the work family, or they seem to spend their best time and energy with the work family, or get harmed by the work family's action or inaction? Ask the family survivor of an officer suicide how they feel about the work "family"? How much is the home family expected to sacrifice for the so-called work family?

Out of respect for our home family, and as a reminder to give our best time and energy to our loved ones, I think we should reserve the word *family* for those precious few who wait for us to return home from work. If compelled to personify and endear the work group, to say with some affection how we feel about our co-workers, I suggest the word *team*. Team seems more fitting and an appropriate distinction between our professional and personal lives. Team members work together towards a common cause, share a purpose and function, and can care deeply about each other.

Once on patrol, I paused when I saw a family, a father, mother, and two small children walking hand-in-hand near a park downtown, a park where I know trouble exists. I wanted any wolves in the area to know the sheepdog was watching. The word *sacred* came to mind, I was witnessing a sacred thing, the family. I do not need to be reminded that families take different forms and that the word *sacred* has a religious connotation, but I saw what I saw and felt what I felt. My purpose as a patrolman in that moment was to protect a sacred thing. We can love police work, care deeply about our coworkers, but the workplace will never love you back in the same way that your family can.

Friends

It may be understandable why cops might exclusively have other cops as friends. Friendships often form around shared interests and values. However, it seems advisable to have non-cop friends, not because cop friends are bad, but because a non-cop identity is good. A non-cop identity can be fostered in many ways, including cultivating other interests and activities.

The difference between acquaintances and friends is that acquaintances require only that you show up, see each other in passing. Relationships with friends, in contrast, need some tending. More is not always better, but we all need a friend or two, people we enjoy and who bring out the best in us. We can have numerous acquaintances, but it seems practically true, as social scientists have suggested, that we can have only so many friends.

Our relationships can be like concentric circles, with our loved ones near us at the center, then friends, acquaintances and coworkers moving outward. We might even consider the outer edges of our relationships to include the repeat criminals who we get to know by being a cop.

Relationships are central to a happy life, not only for a full enjoyable life, but for health and wellbeing as well.

A healthy inner life is interdependent with a healthy outer life. If we want the good life, a happy life, we are compelled to get our hearts right about all the "others" and stay fully engaged with our loved ones and community.

CHAPTER 12

PURPOSE AND FUNCTION

Purpose-Centered Policing

Lean Forward, Stumble Ahead

Early in my public safety career, another paramedic offhandedly said to me, "I wish I could be more like you." At first, I thought he was being a wise guy, mocking me maybe. He was a bit younger, had good hair and drove a sports car. I was married with a new baby, losing my hair and drove a $500 Dodge Omni. Aside from this comment, which suggested that he apparently felt trapped by his desires, my observation of him was that he treated the work like it was easy, yet he was not a particularly skilled paramedic and appeared already bored by the work and was very cynical, as if the job had let him down. To me, life felt like a struggle and I was a blurry eyed new father trying to survive. While he seemed to have the wind at his back, I felt as though I was leaning into it. My sole purpose and function was to move, or at least lean forward in the direction I wanted to go.

Looking back, I was right in the midst of building a good life and did not even know it. If I would have been asked if I were happy, I would have said that I did not know, had not really considered it. I was just trying to make ends meet, get enough sleep, keep a used car running and get good at my job. Like everyone, I was pursuing happiness, but maybe taking the long route. The people I admired were the guys who were really good at their jobs *and* had good hair.

Often, we venture into things with the mistaken belief that it will be easy or with little thought of consequences. Thankfully we do this or we would probably not get married, have children, become cops. Fortunately, there is creativity, which paradoxically cannot be counted on, but sometimes arrives when our plans fail and we must give up or look for an alternative.[1]

Happiness is not our right, but as described by our forefathers, pursuit of it is. Our forefathers spoke of the pursuit of happiness, but did not define happiness for us, instead they sought to guarantee our right to try to achieve it. As adults, the thought of someone else being responsible for our happiness would likely have been laughable to those who have gone before us, and the idea that our work owes it to us would seem absurd. Workplaces get into trouble and leaders fail when the work becomes more about the workers' need for happiness, and less about the work that needs to be done, and when the malcontent worker is allowed to define reality.

If we are honest with ourselves, many of us must admit that we have been the malcontent worker. Which is not all bad, it can be motivation for change, but where we get it wrong is when we blame our unhappiness on the convenient targets, our job, our relationships, and such, but fail to see our part in it. Most often, it has less to do with our job or our relationships, and more (or even all) to do with growing up and maturing. If we are looking to blame our unhappiness on something, it may in large part be due to confusion about our values or spending time and energy pursuing the wrong values.

For some cops, loss of a sense of purpose and function can be a slow and painful death of sorts, revealing itself in such things as absenteeism or showing up for work physically, but not mentally. Take it as a warning that you need to reevaluate your purpose and function if your happiness is dependent on retirement. It seems reasonable that some may count down the last few years, but more than that sounds bleak.

Maturation

Most cops start out young, and work, 10, 20, 30 years, becoming grown men and women in plain view. Discontentment can have little to do with the work of a police officer and have everything to do with maturation, growing up. Not recognizing this is like a missed diagnosis and will make you miserable and unpleasant to be around. Maturation is more about persistence, discipline over luck.

Luck. When I was a child, I could list several things that I and most kids considered lucky or unlucky. The things we did not understand or have control over were best explained as mysteries or magic, failure attributed to stepping on a crack, and advantages sought by crossing your fingers. Lucky rabbit feet were popular, an actual rabbit's foot with a small chain attached, like a key ring, that you could carry in your pocket. Good luck for me was finding money; my specialty was finding coins on the street or in phone booths. I would walk all over town with my head down, never pass a pay phone without checking the change return and pulling the coin release lever. It was not until sometime later that I realized my so-called good luck had more to do with dogged persistence. As a cop, and especially as a patrol supervisor, I considered luck a poor leader, and any reliance on it a danger. We would make our own luck through skill, practice and effort.

Good luck and bad luck may be convenient ways to explain the mysterious or in some cases relieve us of responsibility or effort, but a more mature view of life is that it is full of challenges, and success has a lot to do with persistence and discipline, showing up and trying to make things right.

Discipline. Discipline is not a dirty word and can translate to moment-to-moment contributions to a higher purpose or goal. The word discipline has two meanings in the work world. It can be a formal action to correct someone else's behavior, often we associate this, maybe appropriately as punishment. An example of the first meaning could be a formal documented verbal warning if detention staff find a weapon on your prisoner.

The second meaning is self- or group-training to do certain things in a controlled or habitual way. An example of this meaning of discipline in police work is that every time you take custody of a criminal, you search them for weapons, even if the cop that handed them off to you just did. This kind of habitual behavior is good for everyone.

Persistence. People often fail because they give up at the first sign of trouble or just short of success, when they are 95% of the way there, the first 5% and the last 5% being the hardest. A useful mantra could be, "It's difficult, but do it anyway." And when you suffer a major setback, regroup and find your way again. Upon reflection, our greatest growth was not likely during the good times. Self-doubt, insecurity, feeling bad can be more valuable than unearned confidence. Best to earn your confidence by *doing*, and leave *feeling like it* out of it.

As Winston Churchill said, "Success is not final, failure is not fatal, it is the courage to continue that counts." Difficulties require recovery and regrouping or the discovery of a deeper sense of purpose. This is the difficult but supremely important work of maturation, judged mostly by our actions. Psychologist and author Jordan Peterson advises that we should act in ways that are good for us now, tomorrow and beyond. That we should seek to grow up in ways that are positive for ourselves, our family and everyone else. And if this involves carrying some load, the heavier the better.[2]

Look Around

It is good to look around and consider what you admire about select others. What we notice can be valuable clues to what we long for or possibly find missing in our own lives. Although we can benefit from being cautious of comparing our insides to others outsides, people who are friendly, helpful and supportive can be a great indicator of having healthy and positive inner workings, or in one word, happiness. They are making day-to-day choices that support their wellbeing and have a happy personal life, possibly while managing significant difficulties. Others, some of who might be considered the best examples of "real cops," have the best work stories, but the worst life away from work.

At different periods of our lives we may have admired the "wrong" people, mistook certain actions or traits as real happiness, or failed to see the calm and unassuming people with rich and healthy personal lives, but recognizing our mistaken thinking has value as well.

Who looks happy? Happy and healthy people attract each other, and inversely, negative or malcontents do the same, even to the point of getting fired together. There is no lack of negative people who would love to pull you into their club, to share in their misery. I am not immune to an occasional bitch session or complaint, but it can be like eating fast food: you crave it, devour too much and soon after feel worse for the indulgence. But how can you avoid the temptation? Maybe do what I witnessed one cop do to repel another cop's bitter complaining, he put up his index fingers to form a cross as if trying to ward off a vampire.

Mentors. I grew up in an intact family with dedicated parents and siblings I respected and looked up to. This would rightly be considered a huge life advantage. Yet I still longed for more guidance, mentoring, but never really found it or maybe did not recognize whatever mentoring was there. I think maybe most people feel as if they could have used more help, or maybe in some cases less, meaning they needed more of the right kind of help. I now see that I could have been more deliberate, purposeful in seeking help, and better at recognizing the help that was available but hidden by my pride. Whether it is peer support, interested supervisors, or maybe more importantly a senior officer, we can all do better for each other when we notice distress, missteps or own our longing for receiving or giving guidance. An invigorating option for officers that have been on the job for a long time is to be more active in mentoring younger officers.

Shared purpose. In lieu of mentors, we belong to groups, imperfect as they are. An angry bitter cop once accused me of "drinking the Kool-Aid," or as he put it, "You still believe in the police department." He said it as if I was a fool, and because it was true, it got my attention and caused me to pause, put me back on my heels. I reflected on it and returned to him days later and told him that he was right. I believed in the police department, but not for the reason one might think. It was not because I was completely blind or wanted to climb the ladder, but because I needed to believe that I was part of something good. Ultimately, I recognized the need to believe in something bigger than just myself alone, in a shared purpose.

I have heard officers describe during the bleakest of times, either personal or collective, that their only motivation to do the work is to support the other cops on their shift. Protecting and serving had been reduced to protecting each other. Although I do not imagine this attitude could or should sustain them for months let alone an entire career, it could help a cop through troubled times. I think this speaks to our enduring need for shared purpose and work that has meaning.

Look Inside

Who are you and what do you want? This sounds a lot like what you might say to someone knocking loudly on your door. It is also a question we may ask ourselves, but the answer may be elusive, it evolves as we evolve. Knowing who you are and what motivates you takes some consideration. Cops might find that they do not know what is in their head, how long it has been there, or how it got there. A way to get started looking inside, might be to contemplate a question such as this, "What are the qualities you like least and most in your parents?"[3] Your answers may reveal previously unconscious motivations.

As we evolve, or progress in life, as described by Maslow (physical survival to self-actualization), we move from mostly needs to mostly wants, or maybe they are all needs or all wants, just viewed differently. There are culturally dominant messages of what we supposedly want or need, like more money to buy more things. But we recognize there are some human voids that cannot be filled that way. So, we eventually ask ourselves, "What do I *really* want?"

What do I really want? The more you know who you are and what you want, the less distractions or dissenting views will upset you. Something that has been a particular struggle for many cops, is the recognition of how thin the veneer of trust and respect for police apparently was. The painful realization is that we cannot control the message about what others think or say about us; we cannot make others respect us. If you want something that someone else controls, they control you. The one thing you can control is your self-respect — what you say and think about yourself. This is not as solitary or selfish as it may sound, because self-respect has to do with belonging to something good, having a shared purpose and function, and doing good.

Self and Others. The line between self and others is not so clear when it comes to helping others. Even the most selfless givers receive something. Although, seeking something in exchange may be incompatible with generosity and compassion, givers receive emotions, witness happiness, reach a deeper understanding and feel the love — all the things money can't buy. The experience awakens them to what they desire most.[4]

Relationships. In college I had a professor that had a spark about him which might today be described as emotional intelligence and self-awareness. We were doing some exercise in which we all took turns stating what we most wanted in life. At one point we asked him and were shocked by the answer, he said, "a successful marriage." It was surprising for two reasons; this was a high value we did not expect to come from him for some reason, and because he suggested it was not easy to come by. Committed relationships can be the greatest challenge to personal growth as it generates in us a need to adapt and change for something outside ourselves.

Of all the things that are good and bad for us, turns out that the most important factor for both health and happiness is the quality of our relationships. The Harvard Happiness study showed that close relationships, more than fame and fortune, or any other factor, are the best predictor of happiness.[5] "Taking care of your body is important but tending to your relationships is a form of self-care too."[6] In fact research has shown close relationships "protect people from life's discontents, help to delay mental and physical decline, and are better predictors of long and happy lives than social class, IQ, or even genes."[7]

The *Why*

What is more important: what you do or why you do it? Do you mop the floor or do you clean the floor with a mop? The difference is that the first one can mean just pushing the mop around leaving the floor dirtier than when you started, but the second gets the job done.

Police work is an easy job to do poorly and a hard one to do well. The difference between an effective cop and ineffective cop has to do with the *what*, *how* and *why* of doing the job. The what of being a cop is relatively easy, it only requires that you show up in a uniform. The uniform represents a profession made noble by the *how* and *why* of brave and dedicated cops that have gone before us. If we do the job motivated only by self-interest, we have tarnished the uniform and climbed down off the shoulders of those great cops.

The *how* of being a cop has more variation and a lot to do with how you were raised, trained and held accountable. The *how* allows for creativity, individual style and specialization. The *why* is where the heart is.

I came across a photo of a Minnesota Wild hockey player wearing a Saint Paul Police garrison cap in the team's locker room. This classic police hat has a gold wreath on the front, which has been part of the uniform since the early 1900s. No one routinely wears that cap but a Saint Paul Police officer, especially not a longhaired, bearded, sweaty hockey player. The Wild coach requested the chief provide the cap so the Player of the Game could wear it, this explains the *how*. The coach explained the *why* this way, "It represents determination, grit, leadership and excellence. That's what the SPPD stands for and we are proud to have the men and women who wear the uniform represented in our locker room."

Getting the *why* right, can be a guide to help when things get tough, like when the *what* does not make sense and the *how* is hard to do. I have spoken with cops not long after they held a child who had been shot, waded through a house where an entire family was murdered, volunteered to do death notifications because they felt particularly skilled at it, all of them have described a higher purpose or using the experience to make them better cops, better able to serve some stranger in the future. When we learn the *why*, the *what* and *how* begin to make sense and become more bearable, even a privilege. *(Stories retold with officers' permission.)*

We all are searching for a *why* to the *what*, but this may differ at different times in our lives and career. One or more whys may stay consistent throughout a career, but others may change as well. Cops want and need different things in different stages of their career. Simultaneously, and unrelated to the job, men and women who happen to be cops are going through the different stages of human development.

Putting the *Why* into Words

Many organizations describe their "reason for being" by writing out their vision, values, mission and philosophy. Warriors, soldiers, teams, workgroups, clans and even families, any large or small group united by a common purpose have found a need for a guiding oath, creed, pledge, promise or solemn vow. This serves as a way to unite us during hard times, to guide when the path is unclear, and remind us of our greatest good. We can also do this as an individual.

> *Vision* A person's vision is a description of themselves at some future time. It sets the overall direction for that person, and what the person strives to be. A vision is something to be pursued, it endures and does not change under changing circumstances.

> *Values* These are the collective principles and ideals that guide the thoughts and actions of a person. Values define character, and what a person stands for.

> *Mission* This is a statement that specifies a person's purpose or "reason for being." It is the primary objective of the person's actions. A mission is something to be accomplished.

> *Philosophy* A personal philosophy establishes the "rule of conduct" for that person. It translates the values of the person into a more concrete description of how the values will be applied to daily actions.

A philosophy of life, a promise or an oath will not keep you from harm, but without them, or some guiding principle, it is as if you are lost in the wilderness. Paradoxically, setting limits and boundaries gives you more freedom, directives help you make better choices with more ease.

Protect and Serve

We each swore an oath, but few of us understood its significance at the time or could recall it now. Yet, we are asked to fulfill it with the expectation that we will protect and serve. Whether our squad cars have the phrase *"To Protect and Serve"* on the side or not, the public think they do because they like the idea. That is how many view us, we protect them and come running when they call.

The Romans had a word that may have described this, *virtus* (virtue). The origins of the word *virtus* can be traced back to the Latin word *vir*, or "man." The use of the word began to grow and shift to fit the new idea of what manliness meant. No longer did *virtus* mean a person was a brave warrior, but it could also mean he was a good man, someone who did the right thing.[8] This can be applied further to the men and women of policing, virtuous or striving to be so. The words *protect* and *serve* are not so far off. Exceptions exist, and if we go looking, examples of failure and underachievement, of not always protecting and not always serving well, can also be found. But we do protect and serve as part of our purpose and function, and we do it well in most instances and against great odds. My chief emphasizes "Service with Respect." Our job is to do the public good. It is about service in a way that shows we care.

Personal Mission Statement

Cops work well as a team, we rely on each other. But every cop knows that he or she could suddenly be faced with a situation while alone, with no one to rely on but themselves. Likewise, we can be carried along by the good or bad energy of our coworkers, the common cause of the agency, our profession, but ultimately, we all live in our head and all messages are filtered by our own thinking and beliefs. What guides our thinking and behavior when we are tired, hungry, or pissed off? What guides you when things get difficult?

Cop knowledge and cop skills are not enough to sustain you throughout your career, you additionally need a philosophy to guide your thoughts and actions. Otherwise, you will flounder and find yourself having done something you did not want to do or dwelling somewhere you did not want to be. The surprising benefit of a crisis or challenge or fork in the road is it accelerates the process of clarifying your purpose and function, your philosophy of life. And with clarity, you can act more deliberately.

In Ronald Reagan's first inaugural address on January 20, 1991, he told the story of Martin Treptow, a barber from Iowa, who was killed in France fighting the Germans during the first World War:

> *We are told that on his body was found a diary. On the flyleaf under the heading, "My Pledge," he had written these words: "America shall win this war. Therefore, I will work. I will save. I will sacrifice. I will endure. I will fight cheerfully and do my utmost, as if the issue of the whole struggle depended on me alone."[9]*

As an individualized guide, consider writing a *Personal Mission Statement*. You will find your purpose and function in the place where what matters most to you and what you have complete control over coincide. You can write your own personal mission statement using these rules and answering these questions:

Rules

- Write in terms of your future life and work as a police officer starting today.

- Must be written down.

- Must be a minimum of three sentences long.

- You may not include any "magic words" derivatives of: excellence, quality, best, professional, outstanding, superior, etc.

- You may not use the phrase "go home at the end of the shift" or something similar. You cannot use "safety" as your responsibility to citizens or other cops. The reason for this is that safety is obviously a primary responsibility, and this is asking you to go deeper for your mission statement.

- Because goals or values can conflict, rank them in order of importance.

Write: Answer these essay questions by writing at least one full sentence for each question.

- What is my primary responsibility to the public?

- What is my primary responsibility to the department or agency?

- What is my primary responsibility to other cops?

- How do I know when I am being a good cop?

- What qualities do I admire in others?

Compile these sentences into a short paragraph as your personal mission statement that you keep as a reminder of your why.

I once had a cop tell me a story, which for me was an example of clarity of purpose when faced with difficulty. A man, wild with grief, raged at this officer and her partner about the murder of his daughter. These officers I am sure, represented to the father all those who failed to protect the young woman. The officer responded by saying, "Use me, I can take it." By daily attending to our purpose and function, we can do our duty and withstand whatever is given us. Our integrity and our sense of a higher calling will protect and serve us. *(Story retold with officer's permission.)*

Morale

Cops like to talk about morale being low, and they use it like a sword to slash at the administration. An odd thing about me is I have never been good at detecting if morale is good or bad. A group of cops once tried to impress upon me how low morale was, and I believed them, but checked with the first partner car I ran into and asked them how morale was, they replied, "Morale is good in our car." Meaning, once they got out of the locker room or roll call, things were fine in their squad car, where they controlled the atmosphere. Some agencies, leaders, supervisors, senior officers, and individual cops do yeoman's work to build and sustain good morale, the generalized confidence, enthusiasm, and discipline of a particular group at a particular time. Inversely, some factors can be devastating to morale and some enter into the world of moral injury.

I always felt I had a role in contributing to high morale, in the academy, as a patrolman, an investigator, patrol supervisor and as the EAP Director. It is my belief that it is anyone and everyone's responsibility to contribute to good morale. This is not to say that everything is good and happy, some agencies and workgroups are terribly dysfunctional, and some work environments are miserable, but the only thing each of us ever have is our area of responsibility. I spent my entire adult working career in public safety in urban cities, a constant exposure to dysfunction, but I still enjoyed the work, felt I was contributing to the welfare of others. If I felt burdened by society's failings and needed to fix them, I would have been overwhelmed, instead I did what I could. Tried to play my part well.

We can be more generous in our thinking about what it means to be command staff and administrators, positions that can be additionally lonelier and more isolating. Patrol cops, even the ones that do not like each other, offer some protection, but the further cops are removed from the group the more unprotected they may feel. It is in our DNA that nothing feels better than belonging to the group and nothing feels worse than not.

When I was first promoted and assigned to be an investigator, my new boss stopped by to say hello. I stood with a slightly bladed stance and my hands above my waist. What if I needed to attack him? I had just gotten off the street after years of patrol work. Over time I felt as if I was re-civilizing, patrol cops live in a different world and they should take it as a compliment that the chief and top administrators no longer know what it is like to be a "real cop." Their shoes are on carpet; patrol cops' boots are on concrete, state troopers on asphalt, sheriff deputies on dirt. But the patrol cop may not know what it is like to herd cats or appreciate the reality that the higher one moves up, the less of a cop they are and the more of a politician they need to be.

Cops take pride in saying they hate politics, but we cannot fulfill our human nature without politics, instead we should engage in it. I believe what cops find most distasteful is the mixed message or the top-down mandates that seem illogical, harmful, counterproductive, or in short, dangerous and duplicitous. Underneath the mixed message is often a hidden agenda, or an attempt to be two things at once. The upper ranks and political leaders seem to get themselves into trouble with hypocrisy, and the street cops get in trouble for the lack of it.

Cops have their own misguided agendas, being a deconstructionist (criticizing and tearing stuff down) is easy, try building something or maintaining something as complex as a large police department. Many cops, including myself at times, have complained bitterly about the command staff, and now I see some of my attitudes and expectations were naive and dare I say childish. When a parent is accused of not under-standing the child, the parent cannot help but think, but I was a child and now I am the adult, yet you were never the adult. The command staff can say, but I was a cop and you have never been the boss. It is true that some command staff are in fact predominately self-serving, cowardly, and some may have never really been a "real cop," but everyone has a boss and most just want what the street cop wants, to get the necessary stuff done and stay out of trouble. In many ways it is safer to stay at the bottom and complain about the top.

Cops would do well to be a little less self-centered, and the command staff to be a little more honest about their loyalties and admit the obvious, that although they may wish things could be different, the street cop is not their number one priority, they are number three at best, the agency and the jurisdiction rank higher, as they need be. The harm can come in the mixed message, the forced disingenuousness of pretending otherwise or having two number ones. I believe my agency cares about me, cares about the individual officer, in fact one of the ways they formalize that caring is to have an EAP. What I also know is that they care about the survival of the agency more, and in most ways I am okay with that, our department's survival is dependent on it.

In Defense of Mediocrity

In all my years at the Mediocrity Leadership Institute (that is, any government job I ever had), I learned a lot. There were a number of the mottos: "If a job is worth doing, it's worth doing half-assed. Do not volunteer. Good enough is good enough." I am trying to be funny here, and mediocrity has not been my style, but I do see the logic in it, and the cops I have shared this with have found it helpful, like permission to seek better balance at work for their family's sake. Demonstrating competence and high achievement is often rewarded with more work and responsibility at the same pay. Beyond that gripe, some emotional intelligence could be expressed in the form of a more balanced view of work.

You may have had that experience and paid a price for being an overachiever. While I do not believe balance is always the highest virtue, overinvesting in our work can have negative mental and emotional consequences. The price can be missing out on some joy at home as well as taking the work too seriously and not enjoying the people you work with. There is a price to be paid for poor work to be sure, and in the public safety business, there are times where we must do exceptionally good work, and maybe in some cases, achieve excellence or die trying. But I have some reservations about advising anyone to seek work performance excellence as a routine, or at least the tired old way the word has been used over the last several years, like a motivational con job or mission statement magic talk. In fact, the original meaning of the word excellence may have had less to do with performance and more to do with behaving correctly or moral virtue. In its earliest appearance in Greek, this notion of excellence was ultimately bound up with the idea of the fulfillment of purpose or function, the act of living up to one's full potential.[10]

In every job or responsibility, we can likely identify one or two areas that demand excellence, but broad excellence does not seem sustainable. And it is logistically impossible to continuously add to a priority list without taking something off that list, otherwise the list becomes diluted. I prefer the word *good* or *better* when possible, or maybe I should use a phrase like "not bad." I expect coworkers to be constant contributors and attentive to the work that needs to be done. If you can do excellent work, great, but what should be asked for is good work, over and over again. If continuous excellence is demanded of the police, then the police may demand excellence of the citizenry. Short of that, let us both try to be good cops and good citizens.

The problem with *good* is that is can be confused with *just good enough*. When mediocrity is thought of as self-preservation and used only to keep your spot on the roster, you have achieved what you wanted, very little. Some cops are lazy, doing just enough to not get fired, a few are scoundrels, using the job purely for their own benefit. So being mediocre might be a step up for them. Some should step out, meaning get another job, because police work is too important and it is a great disservice to cause further harm because of your own damage. Supervisory energy and resources are not unlimited. My observation is that it can take an enormous amount of supervisory time and attention to get the low performers to move a quarter-inch while those doing a good job ask for only a little encouragement or the freedom to be left alone. As a supervisor, I want to raise the expectation for good work by all.

As the EAP director, my biggest concern is not for the low performer, or even the good worker, but the high achiever. These I find are the ones that suffer the greatest disillusionment, who can feel the most beaten down by careless mediocrity. My message to the high achievers is, "It's okay to be *just* a good worker." If you are a police officer for one year or thirty plus, be good a lot, rather than try and fail to be excellent all the time. In this case quality goes up with quantity; daily contributions of good can result in a lifetime of excellence. Show up and do the work that needs to be done. High achievers, save your best for your loved ones and seek your excellence away from the job.

Less-Than-Optimal Optimism

I once watched a rabbit seemingly contentedly sniff the nose of a boa constrictor for a full ten minutes before suddenly being devoured. Just as cynicism may not be all-bad, optimism may not be all good and not without its own hazards, especially if you design sky scrapers, fly passenger planes or approach strangers for a living. Constructive pessimism can be vital to building useful ways of thinking. The Stockdale Paradox speaks to this as it relates to survival.

James Stockdale was a POW during the Vietnam War. Stockdale was held prisoner for seven and a half years and tortured routinely. As the senior Naval officer, he was one of the primary organizers of prisoner resistance. Jim Collins interviewed Stockdale and described their conversation in his book *Good to Great*. Stockdale said, "I never lost faith in the end of the story, I never doubted not only that I would get out, but also that I would prevail in the end and turn the experience into the defining event of my life, which, in retrospect, I would not trade."

When asked who didn't make it out of Vietnam, Stockdale replied: "Oh, that's easy, the optimists....Oh, they were the ones who said, 'We're going to be out by Christmas.' And Christmas would come, and Christmas would go. Then they'd say, 'We're going to be out by Easter.' And Easter would come, and Easter would go. And then Thanksgiving, and then it would be Christmas again. And they died of a broken heart." Stockdale then added: "This is a very important lesson. You must never confuse faith that you will prevail in the end — which you can never afford to lose — with the discipline to confront the most brutal facts of your current reality, whatever they might be."[11]

Cops are not in danger of being overly optimistic. Our risk is letting cynicism and pessimism overtake us. What we may need is the middle ground of realistic optimism.

Grand Disillusionment

Many of the things cops instinctually do, like notice suspicious behavior, as well as the things they are compelled to do, are all things society has asked them to do. Cops know the work is necessary and they are able and willing to take the required actions. But every cop also knows humans can be dangerously unpredictable and many do not act as they are asked or told. When an officer closes the gap on a stranger, things can go wrong, and wrong quickly; the result can be unpleasant to say the least. This is doing society's dirty work, and that dirty work becomes the filthiest when that same society now denies they asked for law and order and accuses the police of being the problem. The lowly cop is defenseless. One of the lessons in the academy is when someone brings the fight to you, never be a punching bag, never submit to a beating, because you will be destroyed. Instead you are told, *attack the attacker.* This is not possible when the attacker is the media, people in passing, your own chief or sheriff, elected officials, neighbors, friends and even family members.

This is where cops seem the most harmed, by the grand disillusionment that revealed just how eager many were to believe false narratives about the police, and how vulnerable cops were to being sacrificed for other superficial and shortsighted agendas or calls for passive policing. Moral injury feels like a betrayal, when those who should have or could have shielded you from harm, chose not to. These were the people who knew better, who had experienced otherwise. Instead they stood with those who were overcome by their emotional impulses, or who rejected authority, or who had an interest in escaping accountability for their own actions. Cops treat people individually, and judge them on how they behave (which is more respectful and empowering), often with some generous latitude, even for those who are hostile, because the cop knows how they live, has seen them weep, and knows a bit about their suffering.

A cop's power and might must be restrained, not by avoidance of difficult things but instead by clarity of purpose. It is not good enough to promise support only when the cop does the right thing, the right thing keeps changing, and the wrong thing may have been the best of a lot of other wrong things. If the blind leap is to accuse cops of racism, command staff dishonor themselves and their office by not demanding proof. Some have instead tacitly agreed by sending cops to diversity, inclusion and equity school, where the cops are instructed to judge people by the color of their skin, not the content of their character. Cowardice has its consequences; I believe the greatest law enforcement management failure since Ferguson has been not *speaking power to truth*.

Realistic Optimism

Believing you will be successful is important to achieving success, but also believing it may be difficult is equally important. Do not expect it to be easy. Thinking that simply thinking positive or visualizing success alone will bring success is foolhardy. "Realistic optimists believe they will succeed, but also believe they have to make success happen, through things like effort, careful planning, persistence, and choosing the right strategies. They recognize the need for giving serious thought to how they will deal with obstacles. This preparation only increases their confidence in their own ability to get things done."[12] Unrealistic optimists rely more on wishing, luck, and magic (maybe summarized in the word lazy). At the first sign of trouble they quit, but the realistic optimist expects trouble, some look forward to the challenge.

When I first became a cop I felt very fortunate, and I suspect that when I stop being one I will feel a great loss. In between the beginning and end is our vocation where we can achieve greatness through daily goodness. Contemplate in this very moment what you value most as a cop, your guiding principle and highest priority and in the very moment that follows, act accordingly. If there is confusion, it is because you are unclear about what is in your control with what is outside of your control. Keep it simple, your area of responsibility is your own mind and the reasoned choices that come from it.

We are the good guys, a blessing to a suffering society. We must be careful not to believe or act otherwise. We have gotten enough advice on how to do our job, and we should not be overly influenced by how others define who we are and what we do, but instead we must find our greatest good and stay with it. Let us continue to learn and practice what we do best, law and order, act as guardians and stand between trouble and those needing protection, when necessary, act as warriors. And if we fail big or small, do the next right thing.

For all of us who have worn the uniform, where we saw our vocation in question and have experienced a personal or collective period of disillusionment and grief, if we magically knew it was all going to turn out fine, it would have been easy to endure the criticism, fear, and heartache. But we did not, and we do not, so let us be brave in the unknowing. Let us support each other when it is not easy.

Police work is a craft. The work itself is inherently good, and it requires much more than showing up. We must know that we are servants, and we must serve well.

ROLL CALL

Do Good Work

Roll Call

Police work is probably pretty much the same in most places, a little bit boring, a little bit exciting, dealing with mostly good people going about their lives, occasionally no people exercising the little power they have by being an ass or downright dangerous. And police officers, sheriff deputies, state troopers (I know I missed some) are probably pretty much the same in most places. One difference I suspect is that some cops miss out on the "pre-deployment" group ritual that larger agencies enjoy, the roll call. This is a unique cop experience, being in a room filled with rough men and women preparing to go out and look for trouble. Some are talkers, some doers, some hilariously funny, others pathetic and seemingly retired on-duty, all a potential partner on a call.

When I was a patrolman, a good roll call prepared my mind, a bad roll call was tolerated, such as when told not to smash any more squad cars or remember to add names and phone numbers to reports, when no one wanted to smash a squad car and the dope who did not include a needed phone number should have been talked to directly. But mostly a good roll call was fun.

As a patrol boss, my favorite part of the shift was roll call. I could not wait to see their smiling or angry faces, and I wanted to show them mine. My roll calls started exactly on time with everyone in attendance, and in full uniform because I believed in the psychological benefits of order and predictability, and felt that when on-duty, you should be fully prepared to rush to the aid of someone who needed it. Yet the best roll calls were raucous, rowdy, noisy and irreverent. I understood that I was merely containing wild creatures who were not in their natural habitat as they were better suited for the dark alley than the classroom. My roll calls sometimes included things such as reciting the pledge of allegiance or a chaplain's blessing, a hip hip hooray or three claps for good work or a new baby. I warned them I would not read most memos and be-on-the-look-outs, because they could read themselves and had a duty to prepare. We would review outstanding arrests from our previous shift, starting with, if it applied, why someone was pulled over or considered suspicious in the first place. Also highlighted were the well-written reports, and good, but maybe less dramatic, police work. We might strategize about problem people, properties, or officer safety. Once on Father's Day, we each took turns telling a grandfather story.

I actually prepared for roll call, and by doing so I may have made them appear spontaneous, fun and friendly, yet that was because I valued them and needed to continuously message my priorities. For me, the essential ingredients of a roll call were these: learn something by pointing out recent good police work or bad police work, inspire and have some laughs. I let my disgust and loathing for the predator criminal show, as well as my love for the cops and the work we do.

I focused on the positive as a means of pointing them in the direction I hoped they would go. The negative needed to be put into perspective, and always, they needed reminding of their special purpose and function in society. The only day I was at a loss for words was when twenty first-graders were murdered at Sandy Hook Elementary School, and we felt that somehow, we, though half a country away, had let these children and their parents down.

You Are Okay

I think cops want most to know that they are okay and that they will be okay. While doing police work we can get lost doing what we thought was good. I tell cops that they are going to be okay a lot. One, because I believe it, and two, they need to hear it, and three, it helps to hear it to move them in that direction. There are times when I add qualifiers or warnings because some cops need to know they can make things worse. And if they are not paying attention, they can lose the things they value most. Hope, encouragement and success stories are important, because no matter what someone is dealing with, they need to believe that they can get better.

If you wanted easy work, completely safe work, this is not it. The idea of police work as a calling is an interesting thought, one we may need to revisit in ourselves. I am most disappointed in the cops that have given up on their "naive" desire to *help people*. This is still our job and it can still be done, but maybe helping people is difficult or not as we had originally imagined, requiring readjusting our aim, not abandoning it. If you have any doubt, consider a few examples. A child placement, where you take your time and do your best to reassure them en route to foster care. Or burglaries, where you help the family understand that the burglar was an opportunist, not specifically targeting them. Or you notice someone vulnerable and linger nearby to keep predators away. None of these are dramatic, all of them ordinary parts of the shift, yet powerfully important. We do more good nonchalantly than many get a chance to do well.

As the EAP director, I still do roll call visits and sometimes tell the story of going to our old Detox, which was down a dark damp street near the river. I joke how maybe the drunks we took there thought we were taking them to this lonesome spot to murder them and dump them in the Mississippi. It gets a good laugh. I tell about my first trip to Detox some thirty years earlier when I was a young soft-hearted ambulance attendant. It was my first experience with a down-on-his-luck drunk, a retired schoolteacher who wept saying that he tried to be a good man. At Detox they made him take off his shoes and belt and lie on the floor of a cell. I had felt like crying.

All these years later, and after being witness to much death and destruction, my heartbreak then seems laughable now. But it was new to me then and I did not know what to do with the sights and sounds of grief or sadness. I eventually got good at it, good at not feeling much that is. I am glad for some stoicism, we need it to be grown men and women and to do this work, and we need not feel bad for not feeling bad. I am not asking cops to be more vulnerable at work; they need to protect that soft heart. Instead they can be more purposeful and deal more effectively with their vulnerabilities and their troubles. Most important is that we need not feel numb either, or the other extreme, frightened by our strong emotions. It is when experiences seem stuck or come out sideways, when we isolate for too long, drink too much, or we harm our loved ones with our absence or anger, or our world seems to be getting smaller and smaller, that we should be most concerned. The part of us that notice this is the wise part, serving and protecting ourselves.

Roll ReCall Now that I think of it, cops could also benefit from gathering at the end of each tour, whether formal or informal, led by a patrol boss or senior officer. Cops are men and women who, for a lack of a better term, are domesticated, leave that world and spend a tour working in a sometimes opposite and up-side-down world, and then return again to domestication. As the roll call prepares them for the tour, a roll recall could prepare them for returning home. A cop told me that he had a sergeant that used to send them home with, "Well fellas we tried, we'll try again tomorrow."

A patrol boss or fellow cop may or may not know when a particular tour of duty was rough, disheartening or traumatizing for an individual cop or a whole crew. So, a wise leader might just assume so, and message the following to help them recover before returning to their loved ones: *society asked you to do the work you did today, any emotional pain you suffered for doing it should have its say, let it be felt. And do not be afraid, just notice how it naturally rises, falls, and then fades away. We did not create the suffering; we just had the courage to get close to it. Good police work involves some suffering, as need be. Before we go home, we should pause to feel the results of our righteous duty. We should leave here what we can, so we do not ruminate over what happened or should have happened.* The roll call at the beginning is a reminder of their duty, and the end, a reminder of what they did. In both cases, we can reflect on what we have to be grateful for.

"Disadvantages" Become Advantages

Trust and Control. This struggle with the nature of control helps us see more clearly what is within our control and what is not. As Epictetus stated and authors of The Daily Stoic, elaborated, those that figure out what is within their control, outside of their control, and the in-between "will not only be happier, [but] will have district advantages over other people who fail to realize they are fighting an unwinnable battle."[1]

On Guard for Sudden Violence. With this vigilance we can display fierceness on demand. Where there is trouble, we lean in, hold our ground, and do not retreat. We voice commands, give and receive hard looks. We seek the tactical advantage and take the higher ground. What distinguishes us from thugs is our discipline and our ability to manage our aggression.

These things give us an advantage in life, if we believe as the Roman emperor Marcus Aurelius did, "The art of living is more like wrestling than dancing, because an artful life requires being prepared to meet and withstand sudden and unexpected attacks."[2] We know a lot about what is possible, all the bad things that can happen to people. We can calm our mind by turning back towards center by thinking more in terms of probability, not possibility.

Cynicism, Skepticism, Suspicion. When not taken to the extreme, cynicism, skepticism, and suspicion are ways of thought made useful by seeking evidence and not being overly influenced by superficial things. This is essential for police work, but also helpful as a discerning person.

However, you can be misled by your confidence on occasion, so expand your landscape by both trusting your gut some, but also doubting your thinking some as well. We should view cynicism for what it is, a sometimes necessary tool, an adaptation with some unpleasant side effects. A useful tool on your duty belt, but one best left at work in your locker before you go home.

Estrangement from Society. There is a sting or ache that comes with being estranged from society. Maybe it is the loneliness of being misunderstood or the frustration of being maligned by those whose lives are better because of our presence in society. I conclude that this estrangement may be our chance for our greatest good.

We can choose to think and talk about the suffering we endure as a willing price we pay for the noble work of protecting and serving others. External rewards are fleeting, some unrealized, others unearned, we are better off finding our own rewards. Any suffering and sacrifice that comes with being a blessing to society is more bearable if we do it to meet a responsibility or duty, a higher calling.

Advantages of Being A Cop

On a July night in 2016, I checked on a group of cops, one's badge had been dented, another had a bruised and bloodied face, both had been struck by rocks. One officer showed me her singed pant leg after being struck by an explosive. These were the walking wounded, all still in the fight, who had been on the front line during the largest civil unrest in our city's recent history. Some of the cops were angry, some looked scared, and some had thought they might die.

One cop pulled down his bloody lower lip and showed me his loose teeth. He had hours earlier left his family at a lake cabin to defend the city. Afterwards, I believe, most cops in the department were either glad they were there or wished they had been. There is something about the hardship cops experience, especially as a group, that feels really important, as if it is good for you and good for the group. This led me to think about the advantages of being a cop, to which I have made a partial list.

Direct Experience. Police work is a face-to-face job. Where people call about trouble, and you have to go see for yourself. People flag you down, and you hear them out. You know the actual story that other people only learn about (sometimes wrongly) in the news. It is hard for me to imagine another job where you are involved with such a variety of people, in such a variety of situations.

With this up close and personal experience we test our beliefs about race and poverty, crime and punishment, good and evil. When accused of being the problem, we know better and have tons more direct experience with the issues than those doing the criticism.

Mental and Physical Fitness. The job tests our metal, our temperament. If things get really bad, you probably have a pretty good idea as to whether you will dominate and survive or not. Foregoing pleasure and comfort strengthen us. The mental and physical weight of the uniform alone is a burden. In all weather and all times of day, we are out in the elements with sore feet and a full bladder. The emotional restraint required to endure incessant scrutiny and misguided tirades, while we stay calm, collected and professional exemplifies endurance and strength.

Helping People. Calling for help has never been easier, and we are on the receiving end of 911. When people are afraid, confused or want a wrong to be righted, we arrive and do what we can. Cops will answer that call no matter the trouble or danger. If citizens have a bat or a burglar in their home, they can call us for help.

Realize Gratefulness. In one of his essays, the Roman Stoic philosopher Seneca, said, "Remember that all we have is 'on loan' from Fortune, which can reclaim it without our permission — indeed, without even advance notice."[3] Even upon the slightest reflection, a cop can come up with a long list of things from the last shift worked to be grateful for in their own lives. You see firsthand how quickly and thoughtlessly what people value can be lost. A cop might pause and reflect on this as they return home.

Not everyone gets to be a cop, and we are often made aware of the admiration of those who know they would not or could not. From another perspective, what if you suddenly could not be a cop, some scoff at this as if it would be a great relief; well maybe they are gone already. But many would feel a great sense of loss. The ancient practice of negative visualization, imagining losing what you value, can help a cop return to what they value most in being a cop, or any other area of your life that you apply it to. The result can be less wishful thinking and more gratitude and contentment with what you already have.

Place in History. At any of our agencies, we could find an old black-and-white photo of a cop from years ago, doing the same police activity we are doing today. We are part of a tradition of guardians that dates back more than 2,000 years. We stand today in that long line in history. Many have come before, and there will be many after.

Participate in Ritual. Yunger, who studies soldiers, describes America as a largely de-ritualized society.[4] Not us, we enjoy rituals that begin before our first call. We take on a different persona, affect, demeanor that our loved ones or canine partners notice as we prepare to leave for work. In the locker room, we place on literal armor, and we sit in specific places in the roll call room based on seniority or stature. We leave the safety of our building to do our work guided by routines and good habits so we all will return, remove our armor and go home.

Tribal Nature. We depend on our loyalty to each other and a common cause. We survive by interdependence, as we must watch out for each other maintaining a mental map of where our partners are. It is so instinctual that we may not always notice it. When a cop calls for help, we will stop at nothing to get to them.

We not only dress alike, but we gather at impromptu meetings, huddles and debriefings. My absolute favorite thing about being a patrol cop was standing around after a call and talking, laughing, complaining about whatever. Only cops get to do this and if an "outsider" tries to join in, we will change the subject.

Demonstrate Courage. Just being a cop does not guarantee courage, but it asks for it from patrol officers to command staff, and everyone in between. Each act of courage builds on the next. We should be very careful to not overstate our courage. The courage represented in the uniform was earned by those who went before us, so we must earn it daily or at least not diminish it, or dishonor those who went before us. Real courage comes at personal cost, and unless we are paying that price or expect to pay it, we should be humble.

There is courage in a willingness to pay the price and lock arms with courage. Ask the average person on the street what he would be willing to die for, and he may or may not have a ready answer. Ask a cop in roll call and he probably has an answer, in a large part because he has had to give it some thought, has tested it.

The advantage is that if we know there are things worth dying for, it means there are things worth living for. Our forefathers demonstrated this, the last sentence in the Declaration of Independence, "And for the support of this Declaration, with a firm reliance on the protection of Divine Provence, we mutually pledge to each other our Lives, our Fortunes and our sacred Honor." This is how people talk who are willing to die for a cause.

Discern Good verses Bad (Evil). We are fortunate to know there is a down side, a bad or evil, because with this we realize there is an upside, a good. For those without this knowledge, where everything is relative, everything is flat, there is no hope. We live in hope precisely because we walk between good and evil. In fact, our daily exposure to bad can make us more aware of good, even within ourselves as, "The line dividing good and evil cuts through the heart of every human."[5]

Do Good Work and Be a Force for Good

Police work is not for the meek and requires both armor and agility. Cops survive by their wits. We do our work imperfectly, and if we fail, big or small, we should do the next right thing. When we get our minds right, the sacrifices are welcomed because they have meaning. If we play our part well, live honestly, take responsibility for our own actions, then unquestionable good is our reward. Those rewards are gaining wisdom, developing self-control, participating in justice, and demonstrating courage.

At the end of each roll call I earnestly told the cops they should expect me to do my job well, and I expected them to do their job well. My send-off message was not "Be careful out there." In fact, I preferred more that they be alert than be careful. Instead, I sent them off with "Do good work." We all have a duty to protect our shared purpose and function. For me, *Do good work* has a double meaning, do your job well, and do good. *Be a force for good.*

ACKNOWLEDGEMENTS

I WOULD LIKE TO THANK THE MANY PEOPLE who helped make this book possible:

The men and women of the Saint Paul Police Department, past and present, the finest cops this side of the Mississippi. SPPD is where I learned to be a cop and love being a cop.

Eric who has been a good friend and co-conspirator in truth-telling. He has deepened my understanding of both cops and recovery.

Janet whose skill and dedication to police officers has rightly earned her status as a beloved therapist. Gregg and the other therapists who have served the SPPD well. Ed C., Matt, Wade, Mark and Karen, for their eager support and encouragement. Ed L. for challenging my understanding of mind, consciousness and thought. Three imperfect strangers: Jack, Frank, and Robert.

Jean Cook for her encouragement and insights that added clarity to the manuscript. Maureen Johnson for her expert reading, thoughtful edits and calm professionalism. David Farr for lending his exceptional design eye, patience and years of publication experience.

My in-laws, for their enthusiastic support of my police work. I thank them for all of their encouragement and pride.

My parents, sister and brothers, for the kind hearts they shared with me, and the years of training in ground fighting and real-life applications of justice and order. My family gave me the best advantage in life.

My children, who mostly stayed out of trouble and endured the distinction of being a cop's kid. You have inspired me to be a good man, and I have always known you were my most important success. Every day, each of you makes me proud, each night I look in your direction.

I especially thank Alley Light Press and Teresa who understood best what I was trying to say, sometimes better than I did. Whose editing and book development helped elevate the message and saved the reader from angry rants. This book would not have been possible without her expert help and guidance.

ENDNOTES

Introduction

1. Unattributed due to a lack of clarity about its origin, quoteinvestigator.com/2011/11/07/rough-men/.

2. "Suicide." *Mental Health America*, 2018, www.mentalhealthamerica.net/suicide#ref%2011.

3. *Data & Statistics Fatal Injury Report*. Center for Disease and Prevention (CDC), 2015.

Part I: Health and Wellbeing

1. Anderson, Carl R. "Locus of Control, Coping Behaviors, and Performance in a Stress Setting: A Longitudinal Study." *Journal of Applied Psychology*, vol. 62, no. 4, Aug. 1977, pp. 446–451.

Chapter 1: Cop Think

1. Klay, Phil. *Redeployment*. Penguin Books, 2015.

2. Williams, Kent. "Breach Point: Personal & Professional Breakthroughs for Law Enforcement Personnel." Apr. 2012, Lakeville, Minnesota.

3. "Hypervigilance." *Wikipedia*, Wikimedia Foundation, 13, Nov. 2016, en.wikipedia.org/wiki/Hypervigilance.

4. Caplan, Joel. "Police Cynicism: Police Survival Tool?" *The Police Journal: Theory, Practice and Principles*, vol. 76, no. 4, 1 Sept. 2003, pp. 304–313., doi.org/10.1350/pojo.76.4.304.25821.

5. Scott, Paul John. "The Male Mind - From Worrier to Warrior." *Men's Health*, Dec. 2011, pp. 108–113.

Chapter 2: Stress, Mood and Thought

1. Van der Kolk, Bessel. *The Body Keeps the Score: Brain, Mind, and Body in the Healing of Trauma*. Penguin Books, 2015.

2. Rossman, Martin. "The Healing Mind with Martin Rossman, MD." Public Broadcasting Service (PBS), Aug. 2016.

3. Yerkes, Robert M., and John D. Dodson. "The Relation of Strength of Stimuli to Rapidity of Habit-Formation." *Journal of Comparative Neurology and Psychology*, vol. 18, no. 5, Nov. 1908, pp. 459–482.

4. McGonigal, Kelly. *The Upside of Stress: Why Stress Is Good for You, and How to Get Good at It.* Avery, 2016.

5. Keller, A., Litzelman, et al. "Does the Perception That Stress Affects Health Matter? The Association With Health and Mortality." *Health Psychology*, vol. 31, no. 5, 2012, pp. 677-684.

6. McGonigal, Kelly. "How to Make Stress Your Friend." TedGlobal, June 2013, Edinborough, Scotland. www.ted.com/talks/kelly_mcgonigal_how_to_make_stress_your_friend.

7. Rossman, Martin. "The Healing Mind with Martin Rossman, MD." Public Broadcasting Service (PBS). Aug. 2016.

8. Rossman, Martin. "The Healing Mind with Martin Rossman, MD." Public Broadcasting Service (PBS). Aug. 2016.

9. Rossman, Martin. "The Healing Mind with Martin Rossman, MD." Public Broadcasting Service (PBS). Aug. 2016.

10. Honeycutt, Josh. "8 Tips for Beating Buck Fever." *Quality Deer Management Association*, 27 Oct. 2016, p. 1.

11. "Meditation 101: A Beginner's Guide Animation." YouTube, uploaded by Dan Harris, et al., Happify, 24, Jun. 2015, www.youtube.com/watch?v=rqoxYKtEWEc&feature=youtu.be.

12. "Why Mindfulness Is a Superpower: An Animation." *YouTube*, uploaded by Dan Harris, et al., Happify, 7, Dec. 2015, www.youtube.com/watch?v=w6T02g5hnT4.

13. "Why Mindfulness Is a Superpower: An Animation." *YouTube*, uploaded by Dan Harris, et al., Happify, 7, Dec. 2015.

14. Scott, Paul John. "The Male Mind—From Worrier to Warrior." *Men's Health*, Dec. 2011, pp. 108–113.

15. "Executive Functions | Memory and Aging Center." *UCSF Memory and Aging Center: Dementia and the Brain*, 2018, memory.ucsf.edu/executive-functions.

16. Rossman, Martin. "The Healing Mind with Martin Rossman, MD." Public Broadcasting Service (PBS). Aug. 2016.

17. Gladwell, Malcolm. "The Gift of Doubt- Albert O. Hirschman and the Power of Failure." *The New Yorker*, 24 June 2013, pp. 74–79.

18. Helmond, Petra, et al. "A Meta-Analysis on Cognitive Distortions and Externalizing Problem Behavior." *Criminal Justice and Behavior*, vol. 42, no. 3, 2014, pp. 245–262., doi:10.1177 /0093854814552842.

19. Burns, David D. Feeling Good: *The New Mood Therapy*. Quill, 2000.

20. Beck, Aaron T. "Thinking and Depression." *Archives of General Psychiatry*, vol. 9, no. 4, 1963, p. 324., doi:10.1001/archpsyc.1963.01720160014002.

21. Lloyd, Karen. "Enhancing Emotion Resilience Through Healthy Thinking." Blue Watch Officer Wellness Conference 2018, 4 May 2018, Woodbury, Minnesota.

Chapter 3: Fitness, Exercise and Nutrition

1. Fain, Elizabeth, and Cara Weatherford. "Comparative Study of Millennials' (Age 20-34 Years) Grip and Lateral Pinch with the Norms." *Journal of Hand Therapy*, vol. 29, no. 4, Oct. 2016, pp. 483–488.

2. Yagana, Shah. "4 Simple Ways to Test Your Longevity." *Huffington Post*, 30 May 2014, www .huffingtonpost.com/2014/05/30/longevity-test-_n_5366031.html.

3. Studenski, Stephanie. "Gait Speed and Survival in Older Adults." *JAMA*, vol. 305, no. 1, 5 Jan. 2011, pp. 50–58.

Chapter 4: Sleep

1. Rajaratnam, Shantha M. W., et al. "Sleep Disorders, Health, and Safety in Police Officers." JAMA, vol. 306, no. 23, 21 Dec. 2011, pp. 2567–2578.

2. "Our Cops Are Ticking Time Bombs for Lack of Sleep." *Force Science Institute*, no. 71, 4 May 2007.

3. "Our Cops Are Ticking Time Bombs for Lack of Sleep." *Force Science Institute*, no. 71, 4 May 2007.

4. "Clyde Bartlett Survey." Mark Attridge and Brian Casey, (unpublished) 2016.

5. "What We're Learning about the Science of Sleep." *MPR News*, St. Paul, 28 Nov. 2017.

6. "What We're Learning about the Science of Sleep." *MPR News*, St. Paul, 28 Nov. 2017.

7. "Nevada Department Blesses Napping on Duty with Special Program." *Force Science Institute*, no. 323, 2016.

8. Murray, Brian J. "What Happens in the Brain During Sleep?" *Scientific American MIND*, www.scientificamerican.com/article/what-happens-in-the-brain-during-sleep1/.

9. "What Is Sleep?" *Healthy Sleep*, Division of Sleep Medicine at Harvard Medical School, 18 Dec. 2007, healthysleep.med.harvard.edu/healthy/.

10. McCrabb, Rick. "Expert: There Is No Room for 'Tired Cops'." *Daytondailynews.com*, 1 Sept. 2017, www.daytondailynews.com/news/expert-there-room-for-tired-cops /VkZY4nHJLZRiXUQvSZGawO/.

11. Alhola, Paula, and Paivi Polo-Kantola. "Sleep Deprivation: Impact on Cognitive Performance." *Neuropsychiatric Disease and Treatment*, vol. 3, no. 5, Oct. 2007, pp. 553–567.

12. "What We're Learning about the Science of Sleep." *MPR News*, St. Paul, 28 Nov. 2017.

13. Alhola, Paula, and Paivi Polo-Kantola. "Sleep Deprivation: Impact on Cognitive Performance." *Neuropsychiatric Disease and Treatment*, vol. 3, no. 5, Oct. 2007, pp. 553–567.

14. Peri, Camille. "10 Things to Hate About Sleep Loss." *WebMD*, 13 Feb. 2014, www.webmd.com/sleep-disorders/features/10-results-sleep-loss#1.

15. Reilly, T., and M. Piercy. "The Effect of Partial Sleep Deprivation on Weight-Lifting Performance." *Ergonomics*, vol. 37, no. 1, Jan. 1994, pp. 107–115.

16. Milewski, et al. "Chronic Lack of Sleep Is Associated with Increased Sports Injuries in Adolescent Athletes." *Journal of Pediatric Orthopaedics*, vol. 34, no. 2, Mar. 2014, pp. 129–133. doi:10.1097/BPO.0000000000000151.

17. "Sleep, Performance, and Public Safety." *Healthy Sleep*, 18 Dec. 2007. healthysleep.med.harvard.edu/healthy/matters/consequences/sleep-performance-and-public-safety.

18. Mitler, Merrill M., et al. "Catastrophes, Sleep, and Public Policy: Consensus Report." *Sleep*, vol. 11, no. 1, Feb. 1988, pp. 100–109.

19. "Sleep, Performance, and Public Safety." Healthy Sleep, 18 Dec. 2007. healthysleep.med.harvard.edu/healthy/matters/consequences/sleep-performance-and-public-safety.

20. Mitler, Merrill M., et al. "Catastrophes, Sleep, and Public Policy: Consensus Report." *Sleep*, vol. 11, no. 1, Feb. 1988, pp. 100–109.

21. Rajaratnam, S.M., et al. "Sleep Disorders, Health, and Safety in Police Officers." *JAMA*, vol. 306, no. 23, 21 Dec. 2011, pp. 2567–2578. doi:10.1001/jama.2011.1851.

22. Rajaratnam, S.M., et al. "Sleep Disorders, Health, and Safety in Police Officers." *JAMA*, vol. 306, no. 23, 21 Dec. 2011, pp. 2567–2578. doi:10.1001/jama.2011.1851.

23. Rajaratnam, S.M., et al. "Sleep Disorders, Health, and Safety in Police Officers." *JAMA*, vol. 306, no. 23, 21 Dec. 2011, pp. 2567–2578. doi:10.1001/jama.2011.1851.

24. "Symptoms." *Shift Work Disorder*, 2018, sleepfoundation.org/shift-work/content/shift-work-disorder-%E2%80%93-symptoms.

25. *Healthy Sleep*, 2018, healthysleep.med.harvard.edu/healthy/.

26. "Sleep Studies." *National Sleep Foundation*, 2018. sleepfoundation.org/sleep-topics/sleep-studies.

27. "When to Seek Treatment." *Healthy Sleep*, 2018. healthysleep.med.harvard.edu/healthy/getting/treatment.

28. Clyde Bartlett Survey, Mark Attridge and Brian Casey, (unpublished) 2016.

29. "How Alcohol Affects the Quality-And Quantity-Of Sleep." *National Sleep Foundation*, 2018. sleepfoundation.org/sleep-topics/how-alcohol-affects-sleep.

30. Blahd, William. "The Healing Power of Sleep." *WebMD*, 6 Oct. 2016. www.webmd.com/a-to-z-guides/discomfort-15/better-sleep/healing-power-sleep.

31. Adam, K, and I. Oswald. "Sleep Helps Healing." *British Medical Journal*, vol. 289, no. 6456, 24 Nov. 1984, pp. 1400–1401.

32. "How To Perform the 4-7-8 Breath To Relieve Unhealthy Stress." *DrWeil.com*, 8 May 2018. www.drweil.com/blog/health-tips/a-simple-breathing-exercise-everyone-should-try/.

33. Weber, Tom, et al. "The Connection Between Sleep and Mental Health." *MPR News*, St. Paul, 21 Nov. 2017.

34. Fekedulegn, Desta, and Cecil Burchfiel. "Shift Work and Sleep Quality Among Urban Police Officers: The BCOPS Study." *Journal of Occupational and Environmental Medicine*, vol. 58, no. 3, pp. 66–71.

35. "Coping with Shift Work." *UCLA Sleep Disorders Center*, 2018, sleepcenter.ucla.edu/coping-with-shift-work.

36. Weber, Tom, et al. "The Connection Between Sleep and Mental Health." *MPR News*, St. Paul, 21 Nov. 2017.

37. "What We're Learning about the Science of Sleep." *MPR News*, St. Paul, 28 Nov. 2017.

38. Prichard, Roxanne. "Sleeping Well Through Shiftwork and Stress." Blue Watch Officer Wellness Conference 2018. 4 May 2018, Woodbury, Minnesota.

39. Lammers-Van Der Holst, Heidi M., et al. "Inter-Individual Differences in Sleep Response to Shift Work in Novice Police Officers – A Prospective Study." *Chronobiology International*, vol. 33, no. 6, 2016, pp. 671–677., doi:10.3109/07420528.2016.1167733.

Part II: Harm and Help

1. "Malaise." *English by Oxford Dictionaries*, Oxford University Press, 2018.

Chapter 5: Critical Incidents and Traumatic Events

1. Konnikova, Maria. "How People Learn to Become Resilient." *The New Yorker*, 11 Feb. 2016, www.newyorker.com/science/maria-konnikova/the-secret-formula-for-resilience.

2. Dobbs, David. "Soldiers' Stress: What Doctors Get Wrong about PTSD." *Scientific American*, 1 Apr. 2009, www.scientificamerican.com/article/post-traumatic-stress-trap/.

3. Harper, Yolanda. "The Power of Eye Movements: The ART of Accelerated Resolution Therapy." TEDxUTampa. 30 Mar. 2018.

4. Rogan, Joe, and Sebastian Junger. "Joe Rogan Experience #975 - Sebastian Junger." Episode 975, 9 June 2017, http://podcasts.joerogan.net/podcasts/sebastian-junger.

5. Junger, Sebastian. "How PTSD Became a Problem Far Beyond the Battlefield." *Vanity Fair*, June 2015, www.vanityfair.com/news/2015/05/ptsd-war-home-sebastian-junger.

6. Van der Kolk, Bessel. "Psychological Trauma: Neuroscience, Self-Identity, and Therapeutic Interventions." 27th Annual International Trauma Conference. 1 June 2016, Boston, Massachusetts.

7. "First Responders and Traumatic Events: Normal Distress and Stress Disorders." pp. 1-2., www.traumacenter.org/Resources/pdf_files/First_Responders.Pdf.

8. Siegel, Dan. "Brain Insights and Well-Being." *Dr. Dan Siegel Inspire to Rewire*, 2010, www.drdansiegel.com/blog/2015/01/22/brain-insights-and-well-being-3/.

9. *Use of Force Policy: Dispelling the Myths.* Lexipole, 2017, p. 11.

10. "'Foreign Affairs' To Release 90th Anniversary Issue." *All Things Considered*, National Public Radio, 4 Jan. 2012.

11. Van der Helm, Els, and Matthew P. Walker. "Overnight Therapy? The Role of Sleep in Emotional Brain Processing." *Psychological Bulletin*, vol. 135, no. 5, Sept. 2009, pp. 731–748. doi:10.1037/a0016570.

12. Trafton, Anne, and MIT News Office. "Possible New Weapon against PTSD." *MIT News*, Massachusetts Institute of Technology, 31 Aug. 2015, news.mit.edu/2015/blocking-memory-pathway-prevent-ptsd-0831.

13. Lyadurai, L, et al. "Preventing Intrusive Memories after Trauma via a Brief Intervention Involving Tetris Computer Game Play in the Emergency Department: A Proof-of-Concept Randomized Controlled Trial." *Molecular Psychiatry*, no. 23, ser. 3, Mar. 2018, pp. 674–682. doi:10.1038/mp.2017.23.

14. Everly, George S. *Critical Incident Stress Management (CISM): A Practical Review.* ICISF, 2017.

15. "Acute Stress Disorder." *Traumadissociation.com*, March 28, 2018, www.traumadissociation.com/acutestressdisorder.

16. "Adjustment Disorders." *Traumadissociation.com*, March 28, 2018, www.traumadissociation.com/adjustment.

17. "Posttraumatic Stress Disorder." *Traumadissociation.com*, March 28, 2018, www.traumadissociation.com/ptsd.html.

18. "Video: When Is It Trauma? Bessel Van Der Kolk Explains." *Psychotherapy Networker*, 1 Nov. 2017, www.psychotherapynetworker.org/blog/details/311/video-when-is-it-%20trauma-bessel-van-der-kolk-explains.

19. "Eye Movement Desensitization and Reprocessing (EMDR) Therapy." *American Psychological Association*, July 2017, www.apa.org/ptsd-guideline/treatments/eye-movement-reprocessing.aspx.

20. "Eye Movement Desensitization and Reprocessing (EMDR) Therapy." *American Psychological Association*, July 2017, www.apa.org/ptsd-guideline/treatments/eye-movement-reprocessing.aspx.

21. Shapiro, Francine. *Eye Movement Desensitization and Reprocessing (EMDR)* Therapy. 3rd ed., Guilford Publications, 2001, p. 2.

22. Rosenzweig, Laney. "What Is ART?" *Accelerated Resolution Therapy, 2017,* acceleratedresolutiontherapy.com/what-is-art/.

23. Rosenzweig, Laney. "What Is ART?" *Accelerated Resolution Therapy, 2017,* acceleratedresolutiontherapy.com/what-is-art/.

24. Rosenzweig, Laney. "ART Training." ART Training, 9 Dec. 2017, Brooklyn Center, Minnesota.

Chapter 6: General Mental and Emotion Distress

1. Klay, Phil. *Redeployment.* Penguin Books, 2015.

2. *Adverse Childhood Experiences (ACE) Study.* Centers for Disease Control and Prevention, 2014, www.cdc.gov/violenceprevention/acestudy/index.html.

3. Kierkegaard, Søren, and Alastair Hannay. *The Concept of Anxiety: a Simple Psychologically Oriented Deliberation in View of the Dogmatic Problem of Hereditary Sin.* Liveright Publishing Corporation, 2015.

4. Baddeley, Jenna. "Depression and Its Metaphors Depression: The Common Cold or the Diabetes of Mental Illness?" *Psychology Today,* 3 Nov. 2008, www.psychologytoday.com/us/blog /embracing-the-dark-side/200811/depression-and-its-metaphors.

5. Virzi, Juliette. "25 'Embarrassing' Symptoms of Depression We Don't Talk About." *The Mighty,* 12 Jan. 2018, themighty.com/2018/01/embarrassing-depression-symptoms/.

6. St. Paul Police Department (SPPD) Policy 230.30 Employee Assistance Program, 3, Jun. 2015.

7. St. Paul Police Department (SPPD) Policy 252.00 Employee Assistance Program, 25, Sep. 2017.

8. "Mental Health Problems—an Introduction, Causes." *Mind.org,* 2017, www.mind.org.uk /information-support/types-of-mental-health-problems/mental-health-problems-introduction /causes/#.WrwuoJPwbJM.

9. "Mental Health Problems—an Introduction, Diagnosis." *Mind.org,* 2017, www.mind.org.uk /information-support/types-of-mental-health-problems/mental-health-problems-introduction /diagnosis/#.WrwvUZPwbJM.

10. "Mental Health Problems—an Introduction, Treatment Options." *Mind.org,* 2017, www.mind.org.uk/information-support/types-of-mental-health-problems/mental-health -problems-introduction/treatment-options/#.Wrwv7ZPwbJM.

11. Williams, Kent. "Personal and Professional Breakthroughs for Law Enforcement." Breach Point Consulting. 13 Sept. 2017, Hudson, Wisconsin.

Chapter 7: Behavioral Health Crisis

1. "Major Depression (Clinical Depression)." Edited by Joseph Goldberg, *WebMD,* 9 Apr. 2016, www.webmd.com/depression/guide/major-depression#1-2.

2. Piscopo, K., R. N. Lipari, J. Cooney, & C. Glasheen. "Suicidal Thoughts and Behavior Among Adults: Results From the 2015 National Survey on Drug Use and Health." *NSDUH Data Review,* Sept. 2016. Retrieved from www.samhsa.gov/data/sites/default/files/NSDUH-DR-FFR3-2015/ NSDUH-DR-FFR3-2015.pdf.

3. Lucas, Scott. "Kevin Hines Is Still Alive." *San Francisco Magazine,* 18 July 2013, www.modernluxury.com/san-francisco/story/kevin-hines-still-alive.

4. Rosen, David H. "Suicide Survivors A Follow-up Study of Persons Who Survived Jumping from the Golden Gate and San Francisco-Oakland Bay Bridges." *Western Journal of Medicine,* no. 122, ser. 4, Apr. 1975, pp. 289–294.

5. Friend, Tad. "Jumpers: The Fatal Grandeur of the Golden Gate Bridge." *The New Yorker,* 13 Oct. 2003, www.newyorker.com/magazine/2003/10/13/jumpers.

6. Dao, James, and Andrew W. Lehren. "Baffling Rise in Suicides Plagues the U.S. Military." *The New York Times,* 15 May 2013, www.nytimes.com/2013/05/16/us/baffling-rise-in-suicides -plagues-us-military.html.

7. St. Petersburg College's Florida Regional Community Policing Institute, Center for Public Safety Innovation. *Law Enforcement Suicide Prevention: Training of Trainers. Law Enforcement Suicide Prevention: Training of Trainers,* 2015, pp. 65-66.

8. Klott, Jack. "4-Question Protocol to Use With a Client That's Been Having Suicidal Thoughts." *PESI.com,* 2016, catalog.pesi.com/sq/bh_001119_suicide_email-15920.

Chapter 8: Alcohol

1. "Rehab That Puts Alcoholic Pilots Back in the Cockpit." *CBS News Sunday Morning.*, 12 Dec. 2017.

2. Vaillant, George E. *Triumphs of Experience: The Men of the Harvard Grant Study.* The Belknap Press of Harvard University Press, 2015.

3. "Rethinking Drinking Homepage - NIAAA." *National Institute on Alcohol Abuse and Alcoholism,* U.S. Department of Health and Human Services, www.rethinkingdrinking.niaaa.nih .gov/.

4. *Facing Addiction in America: The Surgeon General's Report on Alcohol, Drugs, and Health.* U.S. Department of Health and Human Services, 2016, Glossary p. 1. addiction.surgeongeneral. gov/sites/default/files/surgeon-generals-report.pdf

5. Wood, Angela M, et al. "Risk Thresholds for Alcohol Consumption: Combined Analysis of Individual-Participant Data for 599 912 Current Drinkers in 83 Prospective Studies." *The Lancet,* vol. 391, no. 10129, 2018, pp. 1513–1523., doi:10.1016/s0140-6736(18)30134-x.

6. Ballenger, James F., et al. "Patterns and Predictors of Alcohol Use in Male and Female Urban Police Officers." *American Journal on Addictions,* no. 20, ser. 1, 8 Nov. 2010, pp. 21–29. doi.org/10.1111/j.1521-0391.2010.00092.x.

7. Clyde Bartlett Survey, Mark Attridge and Brian Casey, (unpublished) 2016.

8. Buettner, Dan. *The Blue Zones: 9 Lessons for Living Longer from the People Who've Lived the Longest.* National Geographic, 2012, https://www.bluezones.com/wp-content/uploads/2015/01 /Nat_Geo_LongevityF.pdf.

9. SAMHSA Center for Behavioral Health Statistics and Quality. "Results from the 2015 National Survey on Drug Use and Health: Detailed tables." 2016, Substance Abuse and Mental Health Services Administration, www.samhsa.gov/data/sites/default/files/NSDUH-DetTabs-2015/NSDUH-DetTabs-2015/NSDUH-DetTabs-2015.pdf.

10. Esser, M. B., et al. "Prevalence of Alcohol Dependence Among US Adult Drinkers, 2009-2011." *Preventing Chronic Disease,* vol. 11, no. E206, 2014. doi:dx.doi.org/10.5888/pcd11.140329.

11. Kessler, R. C., et al. "Lifetime Prevalence and Age-of-Onset Distributions of DSM-IV Disorders in the National Comorbidity Survey Replication." *Archives of General Psychiatry,* vol. 62, no. 6, 2005, pp. 593-602.

12. Facing Addiction in America: *The Surgeon General's Report on Alcohol, Drugs, and Health.* U.S. Department of Health and Human Services, 2016, Ch 2, p.3. addiction.surgeongeneral.gov /sites/default/files/surgeon-generals-report.pdf.

13. American Psychiatric Association. (2013). *Diagnostic and Statistical Manual of Mental Disorders (DSM5) (5th ed.).* Arlington, VA: American Psychiatric Publishing.

14. *Facing Addiction in America: The Surgeon General's Report on Alcohol, Drugs, and Health.* U.S. Department of Health and Human Services, 2016, Ch 1, p. 16. addiction.surgeongeneral. gov/sites/default/files/surgeon-generals-report.pdf.

15. SAMHSA Center for Behavioral Health Statistics and Quality. "Results from the 2015 National Survey on Drug Use and Health: Detailed tables." 2016, Substance Abuse and Mental Health Services Administration, ww.samhsa.gov/data/sites/default/files/NSDUH-DetTabs-2015 /NSDUH-DetTabs-2015/NSDUH-DetTabs-2015.pdf.

16. *Facing Addiction in America: Surgeon General's Report,* 2016, Ch. 1, p. 1. addiction .surgeongeneral.gov/sites/default/files/surgeon-generals-report.pdf.

17. *Facing Addiction in America: Surgeon General's Report,* 2016, Ch. 1, p. 2.

18. United States, Congress, Division of Population Health. "Alcohol and Public Health." *CDC. gov,* June 2017. www.cdc.gov/alcohol/data-stats.htm.

19. *Facing Addiction in America: Surgeon General's Report,* 2016, Ch. 2, p. 7. addiction. surgeongeneral.gov/sites/default/files/surgeon-generals-report.pdf.

20. *Facing Addiction in America: Surgeon General's Report,* 2016, Ch. 2, p. 8.

21. *Facing Addiction in America: Surgeon General's Report,* 2016, Ch. 2, p. 8.

22. *Facing Addiction in America: Surgeon General's Report,* 2016, Ch. 2, p. 4.

23. *Facing Addiction in America: Surgeon General's Report,* 2016, Ch. 2, p. 6.

24. Ball, G., Stokes, et al. "Executive Functions and Prefrontal Cortex: A Matter of Persistence?" *Frontiers in Systems Neuroscience,* vol. 5, no. 3, 2011, pp. 1-13.

25. *Facing Addiction in America: Surgeon General's Report*, 2016, Ch. 2, p. 2. addiction. surgeongeneral.gov/sites/default/files/surgeon-generals-report.pdf.

26. *Facing Addiction in America: Surgeon General's Report*, 2016, Ch. 2, p. 6.

27. *Facing Addiction in America: Surgeon General's Report*, 2016, Ch. 2, p. 10.

28. *Facing Addiction in America: Surgeon General's Report*, 2016, Ch. 2, pp. 12-13.

29. *Facing Addiction in America: Surgeon General's Report*, 2016, Ch. 2, pp. 12-13.

30. Koob, G. F., & M. Le Moal. "Drug Addiction, Dysregulation of Reward, and Allostasis." *Neuropsychopharmacology*, vo. 24, no. 2, 2001, pp. 97-129.

31. *Facing Addiction in America: Surgeon General's Report*, 2016, Executive Summary p.5-6. addiction.surgeongeneral.gov/sites/default/files/surgeon-generals-report.pdf.

32. *Facing Addiction in America: Surgeon General's Report*, 2016, Ch. 2, pp. 17-18.

33. *Facing Addiction in America: Surgeon General's Report*, 2016, Ch. 2, p. 18.

34. *Facing Addiction in America: Surgeon General's Report*, 2016, Ch. 2, p. 23.

35. Anthenelli, R. M. "Focus on: Comorbid Mental Health Disorders." *Alcohol Research & Health*, vol. 33, no. 1-2, 2010, pp. 109-117.

36. Holmes, A., et al. "Chronic Alcohol Remodels Prefrontal Neurons and Disrupts NMDAR-Mediated Fear Extinction Encoding." *Nature Neuroscience*, vol. 15, no. 10, 2012, pp. 1359-1361.

37. *Facing Addiction in America: Surgeon General's Report*, 2016, Ch. 2, p. 23. addiction. surgeongeneral.gov/sites/default/files/surgeon-generals-report.pdf.

38. Ball, G., et al. "Executive Functions and Prefrontal Cortex: A Matter of Persistence?" *Frontiers in Systems Neuroscience*, vol. 5, no. 3, 2011, pp. 1-13.

39. *Facing Addiction in America: Surgeon General's Report*, 2016, Ch. 4, p. 15. addiction. surgeongeneral.gov/sites/default/files/surgeon-generals-report.pdf.

40. *Facing Addiction in America: Surgeon General's Report*, 2016, Ch. 4, pp. 12-13.

41. *Facing Addiction in America: Surgeon General's Report*, 2016, Ch. 4, pp 29-29.

42. *Facing Addiction in America: Surgeon General's Report*, 2016, Ch. 5, p. 8.

43. *Facing Addiction in America: Surgeon General's Report*, 2016, Executive Summary p.10.

44. *Facing Addiction in America: Surgeon General's Report*, 2016, Ch. 4, p. 14.

45. White, W. L. "Recovery/remission from substance use disorders: An analysis of reported outcomes in 415 scientific reports, 1868-2011." Philadelphia, PA: Philadelphia Department of Behavioral Health and Intellectual Disability Services, 2012, www.naadac.org/assets/1959/whitewl2012_recoveryremission_from_substance_abuse_disorders.pdf.

46. *Facing Addiction in America: Surgeon General's Report*, 2016, Ch. 5, p. 2. addiction. surgeongeneral.gov/sites/default/files/surgeon-generals-report.pdf.

47. *Facing Addiction in America: Surgeon General's Report*, 2016, Ch. 5, p. 10.

48. *Facing Addiction in America: Surgeon General's Report*, 2016, Ch. 5, p. 10.

49. Kaskutas, L. A., et al. "Elements That Define Recovery: The Experiential Perspective." *Journal of Studies on Alcohol and Drugs*, vol. 75, no. 6, 2014, pp. 999-1010.

50. *Facing Addiction in America: Surgeon General's Report*, 2016, Ch. 7, pp. 16-17. addiction. surgeongeneral.gov/sites/default/files/surgeon-generals-report.pdf.

51. *Facing Addiction in America: Surgeon General's Report*, 2016, Ch. 2, p. 2.

52. *Facing Addiction in America: Surgeon General's Report*, 2016, Ch. 3, pp. 4-5.

53. *Facing Addiction in America: Surgeon General's Report*, 2016, Ch. 3, p. 4-7.

54. DiClemente, C. C., S. K. Fairhurst, & N. A. Piotrowski. "Self-Efficacy and Addictive Behaviors." *Self-Efficacy, Adaptation, and Adjustment: Theory, Research and Application.* Edited by James E. Maddux, Springer, 1995, pp. 109-141.

55. Locke, E. A., E. Frederick, C. Lee, & P. Bobko. "Effect of Self-Efficacy, Goals, and Task Strategies on Task Performance." *Journal of Applied Psychology*, vol.69, no. 2, 1984, pp. 241-251.

56. *Facing Addiction in America: Surgeon General's Report*, 2016, Ch. 4, p. 4. addiction .surgeongeneral.gov/sites/default/files/surgeon-generals-report.pdf.

57. Mockovak, Milan. "The Accountable Supervisor." 2014, St. Paul, Minnesota.

58. "Rehab That Puts Alcoholic Pilots Back in the Cockpit." *CBS News Sunday Morning.*, 12 Dec. 2017.

59. "Work-Life Reference Materials." *U.S. Office of Personnel Management*, 2018, www.opm.gov /policy-data-oversight/worklife/reference-materials/alcoholism-in-the-workplace-a-handbook -for-supervisors/.

Chapter 9: Struggle and Change

1. Mineo, Liz. "Good Genes Are Nice, but Joy Is Better." *The Harvard Gazette*, 11 Apr. 2017, news. harvard.edu/gazette/story/2017/04/over-nearly-80-years-harvard-study-has-been-showing -how-to-live-a-healthy-and-happy-life/.

2. Quote by Winston Churchill, post-war years (1945-1955) As cited in *The Forbes Book of Business Quotations* (2007), Ed. Goodwin, Black Dog Publishing, p. 168.

3. Unattributed due to a lack of clarity about its origin, quoteinvestigator.com/2010/07/14/luck/.

4. "Struggle For Smarts? How Eastern And Western Cultures Tackle Learning." *Morning Edition*, NPR, 12 Nov. 2012. www.npr.org/sections/health-shots/2012/11/12/164793058/ struggle-for-smarts-how-eastern-and-western-cultures-tackle-learning.

5. "Struggle For Smarts? How Eastern And Western Cultures Tackle Learning." *Morning Edition*, NPR, 12 Nov. 2012. www.npr.org/sections/health-shots/2012/11/12/164793058/ struggle-for-smarts-how-eastern-and-western-cultures-tackle-learning.

6. Williams, Hank. "I'm So Lonesome I Could Cry." Heerzog Studio, Cincinnati, OH, 8 Nov. 1949.

7. "'I Saw The Light' Takes Actor Back To Classical Roles." *Weekend Edition Sunday*, NPR, 27 Mar. 2016, www.npr.org/2016/03/27/472035945/i-saw-the-light-takes-actor-back-to-classical-roles.

8. Jung, C. G. *The Undiscovered Self.* Signet, 2006.

9. Brooks, David, "Opinion: What Suffering Does." The New York Times, 7 Apr. 2015, www .nytimes.com/2014/04/08/opinion/brooks-what-suffering-does.html.

10. Quote by Louis Pasteur.

11. Scott, Paul John, and Peter Hapak. "From Worrier to Warrior." *Men's Health*, 17 Nov. 2011, p. 114. Kristen Ellard.

12. Quote by Raj Beekie.

13. Konnikova, Maria. "How People Learn to Become Resilient." *The New Yorker*, 11 Feb. 2016, www.newyorker.com/science/maria-konnikova/the-secret-formula-for-resilience.

14. Reivich, Karen, & Andrew Shattel. *The Resilience Factor: 7 Keys to Finding Your Inner Strength and Overcoming Life's Hurdles.* Broadway Books, 2003.

15. Konnikova, Maria. "How People Learn to Become Resilient." *The New Yorker*, 11 Feb. 2016, www.newyorker.com/science/maria-konnikova/the-secret-formula-for-resilience.

16. Konnikova, Maria. "How People Learn to Become Resilient." *The New Yorker*, 11 Feb. 2016.

17. Konnikova, Maria. "How People Learn to Become Resilient." *The New Yorker*, 11 Feb. 2016.

18. Anderson, Carl R. "Locus of Control, Coping Behaviors, and Performance in a Stress Setting: A Longitudinal Study." *Journal of Applied Psychology*, 62(4), Aug. 1977, pp. 446–451.

19. Konnikova, Maria. "How People Learn to Become Resilient." *The New Yorker*, 11 Feb. 2016.

20. Konnikova, Maria. "How People Learn to Become Resilient." *The New Yorker*, 11 Feb. 2016.

21. Konnikova, Maria. "How People Learn to Become Resilient." *The New Yorker*, 11 Feb. 2016.

Chapter 10: Peer Support and Early Intervention

1. Epictetus. *Handbook*, 16.

2. "Paul Bloom: Against Empathy: The Case for Rational Compassion." *YouTube*, uploaded by Carnegie Council for Ethics in International Affairs, Dec. 2016, www.youtube.com/ watch?v=yhCGmDJQRpc.

3. Voegeli, William. "The Case Against Liberal Compassion." *Hillsdale College Imprimis*, vol. 43, ser. 10, Oct. 2014. imprimis.hillsdale.edu/the-case-against-liberal-compassion/.

4. Junger, Sebastian. "How PTSD Became a Problem Far Beyond the Battlefield." *Vanity Fair*, June 2015, www.vanityfair.com/news/2015/05/ptsd-war-home-sebastian-junger.

5. Junger, Sebastian. "How PTSD Became a Problem Far Beyond the Battlefield." *Vanity Fair*, June 2015.

6. Junger, Sebastian. "How PTSD Became a Problem Far Beyond the Battlefield." *Vanity Fair*, June 2015.

7. "Peer Support: Research and Reports." *Mental Health America*, 24 Jan. 2018, www
.mentalhealthamerica.net/conditions/peer-support-research-and-reports.

8. "Value of Peers, 2017." *Mental Health America*, SAMHSA, www.samhsa.gov/sites/default/
files/programs_campaigns/brss_tacs/value-of-peers-2017.pdf.

9. Headlee, Celeste. "10 Ways to Have a Better Conversation." *TEDxCreativeCoast*, May 2015,
www.ted.com/talks/celeste_headlee_10_ways_to_have_a_better_conversation.

10. Stafford, William. "With Kit, Age 7, At The Beach" *The Rag and Bone Shop of the Heart:
Poems for Men*, edited by Robert Bly, James Hillman, and Michael Meade, HarperCollins, 1993,
pp. 33-37.

11. Stafford, William. "With Kit, Age 7, At The Beach" *The Rag and Bone Shop of the Heart:
Poems for Men*, edited by Robert Bly, James Hillman, and Michael Meade, HarperCollins, 1993,
pp. 33-37.

12. Stafford, William. "With Kit, Age 7, At The Beach" *The Rag and Bone Shop of the Heart:
Poems for Men*, edited by Robert Bly, James Hillman, and Michael Meade, HarperCollins, 1993,
pp. 33-37.

13. Taranowski, Chester J., & Kathleen M. Mahieu. "Trends in Employee Assistance Program
Implementation, Structure, and Utilization, 2009 to 2010." *Journal of Workplace Behavioral
Health*, vol. 28, no. 3, 7 Aug. 2013, pp. 172–191. doi.org/10.1080/15555240.2013.808068.

14. Blue Light Programme—Support for Emergency Services, www.mind.org.uk/bluelight.

Part III: Thrive

Chapter 11: Inner Life and Outer Life

1. Baggini, Julian. "Wisdom's Folly: The Unexamined Life Is Not Worth Living, Plato." *The
Guardian*, Guardian News and Media, 12 May 2005, www.theguardian.com/theguardian/2005
/may/12/features11.g24.

2. Neff, Kristin & Christopher Germer. "Self-Compassion and Psychological Well-Being."
The Oxford Handbook of Compassion Science, edited by Emma Seppala et al., Oxford University
Press, 2017.

3. Unattributed due to a lack of clarity about its origin, aharon.varady.net/omphalos/2016/04
/first-said-forgiveness-giving-hope-better-past.

4. Williamson, Marianne. *A Return to Love: Reflections on the Principles of A Course in
Miracles*. HarperPerennial, 1992, p. 51.

5. McGarvey, Bill. "Our Nation's Greatest Contribution to Religious Thought Is Alcoholics
Anonymous." *America—The Jesuit Review*, 12 Oct. 2016, www.americamagazine.org/politics
-society/2016/10/12/our-nations-greatest-contribution-religious-thought-alcoholics.

6. Epictetus, and Sharon Lebell. The Art of Living the Classic Manual on Virtue, Happiness,
and Effectiveness. HarperSanFrancisco, 1995.

7. Neiburhr, Reinhold. "The Serenity Prayer." Complete, Unabridged, Original Version,
en.wikipedia.org/wiki/Serenity_Prayer.

Chapter 12: Purpose and Function

1. Gladwell, Malcolm. "The Gift of Doubt- Albert O. Hirschman and the Power of Failure."
The New Yorker, 24 June 2013, pp. 74–79.

2. Peterson, Jordan. Jordan Peterson Online Video Collection, 2017.

3. Bryant, Adam. "The New York Times." 27 Oct. 2017. Interview with Bob Brennan.

4. "Why Do Some People Go out of Their Way to Help Others?" *YouTube*, uploaded by Lap Lap
Chap Chap, 1 Mar. 2016, www.youtube.com/watch?v=HJjZ4ZU5f-g.

5. Mineo, Liz. "Good Genes Are Nice, but Joy Is Better." *The Harvard Gazette*, 11 Apr. 2017,
news.harvard.edu/gazette/story/2017/04/over-nearly-80-years-harvard-study-has-been
-showing-how-to-live-a-healthy-and-happy-life/.

6. Mineo, Liz. "Good Genes Are Nice, but Joy Is Better." *The Harvard Gazette*, 11 Apr. 2017.

7. Mineo, Liz. "Good Genes Are Nice, but Joy Is Better." *The Harvard Gazette*, 11 Apr. 2017.

8. "Virtus (Virtue)." *Wikipedia*, Wikimedia Foundation, 12 Apr. 2018, en.wikipedia.org/wiki
/Virtus_(virtue).

9. Ronald Reagan: "Inaugural Address," January 20, 1981. Online by Gerhard Peters and John T. Woolley, *The American Presidency Project*. http://www.presidency.ucsb.edu/ws/?pid=43130.

10. "Arete (Moral Virtue)." *Wikipedia*, Wikimedia Foundation, 12 Apr. 2018, en.wikipedia.org /wiki/Arete_(moral_virtue).

11. Collins, Jim *Good to Great*. Harper Business, 2001, pp. 87-88.

12. Grant, Heidi. "Managing Yourself: Be an Optimist Without Being a Fool." *Harvard Business Review*, 2 May 2011, hbr.org/2011/05/be-an-optimist-without-being-a.

Conclusion: Roll-Call

1. Holiday, Ryan, and Stephen Hanselman. *The Daily Stoic: 366 Meditations on Wisdom, Perseverance, and the Art of Living*. Portfolio/Penguin, 2016, p 9.

2. Marcus, VII. 61.

3. Seneca. "To Marcia," I.7, IX.2, X.3.

4. Junger, Sebastian. "How PTSD Became a Problem Far Beyond the Battlefield." *Vanity Fair*, June 2015, www.vanityfair.com/news/2015/05/ptsd-war-home-sebastian-junger.

5. Solzhenitsyn, Alexander Isaevich, "The Bluecaps." *The Gulag Archipelago: 1918-1956: An Experiment in Literary Investigation, 1918-1956*. Collins and Harvill, 1974, p. 168.

INDEX

ABOUT THE AUTHOR

BRIAN CASEY is a sergeant at the Saint Paul Police Department and director of their Employee Assistance Program. He has a degree in Health Education from the University of Minnesota and over thirty years experience working as a paramedic, EMS Educator and police officer. His personal experience with critical incidents and his work as a health educator have given him special insight into the health and wellbeing of public safety personnel.